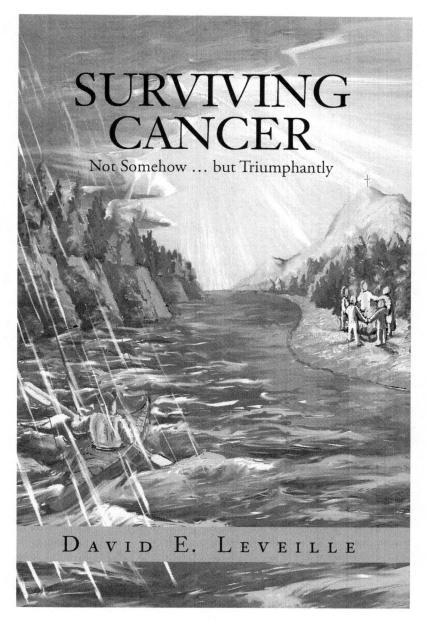

SURVIVING CANCER

Not Somehow ... but Triumphantly

DAVID E. LEVEILLE

WESTBOW
PRESS
A DIVISION OF THOMAS NELSON
& ZONDERVAN

WestBow Press books may be ordered through booksellers or by contacting:

WestBow Press
A Division of Thomas Nelson & Zondervan
1663 Liberty Drive
Bloomington, IN 47403
www.westbowpress.com
1 (866) 928-1240

ISBN: 978-1-4908-2555-7 (sc)
ISBN: 978-1-4908-2556-4 (hc)
ISBN: 978-1-4908-2554-0 (e)

Library of Congress Control Number: 2014902256

Printed in the United States of America.

WestBow Press rev. date: 02/13/2014

Author's Note

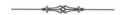

The graphic, beautifully designed by my daughter, Michelle, reflects my experiences from the time of being diagnosed with cancer to the present day and hopefully into the future.

It depicts a vision of me paddling upstream through rough waters, going onward and upward in what at times was for me a battle against the odds. The turbulence of the waters and the storm clouds overhead are intended to reflect my initial thinking at the outset of the journey.

I share with Ralph Waldo Emerson a deep and abiding reverence for water. It is, for me, a source of strength, refreshment, and rejuvenation. Probably the most pervasive image throughout Emerson's writings is the image of water. Water's fluidity, its clarity, and its shapeless character seem to have fascinated him. Water has several meanings, all of which relate to basic concepts associated with independence, transcendence, and spiritual insight.

In his 1836 essay, *Nature*, Emerson asks, "Who looks upon a river in a meditative hour and is not reminded of the flux of all things." The flowing river not only reminds me of the ongoing flow of time; it is also a figure for the passing days of an individual's life.

In "The Over-Soul," another essay by Emerson first published in 1841, in which images of water also abound, he writes, "Man is a stream whose source is hidden," a statement that emphasizes the mystery he finds in each person.

The raindrops are illustrative of the "crushed ice" experience depicted in the narrative of the book. Rain is meaningful to me. It brings out a sense of melancholy, a time of reflection, and always a time to think about God. When our lives feel thirsty and dry, it is the rain that comes to quench that thirst. At times it is clothed in pain and sorrow, and its mantle feels heavy on our shoulders. Still the fresh water that is poured between the cracks and rocky places flows deep into the rich, warm soil of our hearts. It then brings healing to our brokenness as our earth mends itself with the gift it has been given. Rain—and water via the "crushed ice"—set me on a course toward opportunities that came my way.

Over on the side are prayer warriors, many known and many others not known directly, who raised their voices in multiple ways not only to lift my spirits but also to minister medically to my body. Just as smiling and talking to people at a party builds connections and relationships, so does praying for others. When one person prays for others, the person praying is more likely to think of others, take the time to listen to them, and be a part of their lives. Offering others support and encouragement can deepen relationships and give people a sense of meaning and purpose separate from themselves and their own lives. When one person says a prayer for someone else, it can benefit both people. It did in my case.

Ahead on this journey the *clouds* began to lift, and then the sun shone brightly. My heart and mind—my very soul—were lifted to a higher place, and I was able to have an out-of-body engagement, in part through my mind but also through the transformative experiences I had on this continuing journey.

The mountaintop provides a vision of the future. My vision of the future is also one of glory, one of a Christ who has ascended into heaven and sits at the right hand of God. It is a wonderful future that is proclaimed by my Christian faith. And it is a future I trust shall come to pass.

To my wonderful wife, Marty, who makes me whole!

Contents

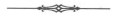

Introduction

This book chronicles a sixteen-year period—my cancer journey. Within my compulsion to tell this story in detail lies the hope of benefiting others, whether the reader is a patient, family member, or caregiver. Cancer affects every person at least once in his or her life in one way or another. Some of the information included is intended to be practical, some spiritual, and all of it personal. Although each situation is different, there is a strong tie that develops among sufferers from the similarities of this dreaded disease and a bond that evolves unlike any other through the encouragement, experiences, and support of others. That is undoubtedly why cancer patients who participate in cancer support groups have a 30 percent improved survival rate. Without exception, these are *people who truly understand what it means to fight the battle against cancer.* Unquestionably knowledge is power, and that includes the volumes of material available on every aspect of cancer. Individual values, a relationship with God, and hope for the future are also big parts of the decisions made. Cancer is no longer a death sentence, but the avenues to restoring health are dependent on choices an individual makes *in combination* with medical professionals.

My ultimate hope and prayer is that I might help you survive and be victorious over the disease, whether you are dealing with it or you know someone who has it. I hope that you will achieve that "peace that surpasses all understanding."

Preface

To every thing there is a season, and a time
to every purpose under the heaven:
A time to be born, and a time to die; a time to plant,
and a time to pluck up that which is planted;
A time to kill, and a time to heal; a time to
break down, and a time to build up;
A time to weep, and a time to laugh; a time
to mourn, and a time to dance;
A time to cast away stones, and a time to gather stones together;
a time to embrace, and a time to refrain from embracing;
A time to get, and a time to lose; a time
to keep, and a time to cast away;
A time to rend, and a time to sew; a time to
keep silence, and a time to speak;
A time to love, and a time to hate; a time
of war, and a time of peace.

—Ecclesiastes 3:1–8

Each year in the United States more than sixty-two thousand people are diagnosed with melanoma. There are an estimated 723,000 melanoma survivors living in the United States today.

Add one to the number.

Me.

More than two million men in the United States count themselves as prostate cancer survivors.

Add one to the number.

Me.

I am told that I am a miracle in this continuing saga.

What a journey! What a blessing! What a life! And there's more to come!

It has been said that cancer is a name and not a death sentence. I concur with that assessment, but cancer really sucks.

On April Fools' Day in 1997, my experience with melanoma began. I had surgery to remove a growth on the top of my head. Life went on with monitoring by my dermatologist and without incident until 2002. The melanoma reappeared, and I had surgery in the same area of my head. Three years after that in May 2005, my normal life took a backseat. Another biopsy from the same area—the top of my head—revealed that I had stage-four melanoma. First my dermatologist and then my oncologist told my wife, Marty, who had remained steadfast by my side, and said that my time on earth was short unless a successful intervention occurred.

Metastatic melanoma is a very challenging disease to treat, and there have been no significant therapeutic advances in the past twenty years. (However, in August 2010 a new targeted drug called PLX4032 was announced by investigators at Memorial Sloan-Kettering Cancer Center and colleagues at other cancer centers. Researchers say that the treatment inhibits the genetic BRAF protein and shuts off these tumors.)

I have had to face my own fears and find out more deeply what I really believed about myself as well as my character. Since I was diagnosed with cancer, I have found one of the most important things that determines my outcome is the kind of person I am and how I respond. Until I faced cancer—or for that matter any other of life's challenges—I really did not know how I would react as a result.

It has also been my experience that, as difficult as it can be to deal with cancer, it can be a blessing in disguise.

Cancer can be a teacher, a hard teacher but an effective one. If you are willing to humble yourself and commit yourself, cancer can teach you profound lessons.

Cancer is also a journey. Each person takes his or her own pathway, and there are many routes on the way. Though the path for many has been well worn by those who have experienced similar struggles, there are also new avenues those willing to deal with the risk of pursuing the unknown can develop. I have been very fortunate in my own way. Many have shared their encounters with cancer with me. No one asks for the battles with cancer, but many of the individuals I have had the opportunity to meet have had courage and a fighting spirit that deserve our applause.

My medical team and fellow patients have been an inspiration. My faith has been strong and has surpassed my own understanding. My family has been there for me every step of the way, serving multiple roles in this sometimes lonely passage. Real friends have stuck with me, and new ones have inspired me and lifted my spirits with daily comments, humor, and kinship that I had not experienced before.

During my journey with melanoma and prostate cancer I have had enthusiastic, compassionate support. Marty insisted I become involved in The Wellness Community, now the Cancer Support Community, a group that has dedicated itself for more than twenty-five years to addressing the issues of quality of life and the fight for recovery. I was reluctant to become a part of this or any other group experience. I don't see myself as a groupie, and I am very private person. That all changed as time progressed and other participants took me in as a part of the community. By opening up their lives to me and to one another, they have given me gifts that can't be adequately described in words. We *care* for one another!

Members of the Cancer Support Community are the pacesetters on a track that leads the way to the healing process for those we honor and love. There is no place for false hope. The victory lap begins and ends in the mind as well as in the heart and soul. The fact remains, however, that the engagement with cancer is not over yet. I remain a work in progress, not only as it relates to cancer but also as it relates to my development as a person. This fact has been underscored by a longtime dear friend and my dentist, Dr. Marlene Schultz. Repeatedly she has said to me, "Dave, God is not through with you yet, and you have many more things to accomplish in this life."

Cancer affects the whole person, not just the area of the body where it resides. As such, cancer responds best to an approach that treats the whole person—body, mind, and spirit. As patients, we do best if we actively involve ourselves in all aspects of our treatment. This book is the fruit of my active engagement in my experiences with cancer and the *power* available to me and to others engaged in their own rendezvous with cancer. Sharing what I learned of myself is my motivation for writing this book, relating my story from the inception of my cancer diagnosis to the present.

After multiple challenges I am now enjoying my family and friends. The arena of cancer is more than difficult for those who have the disease and for all those who care for the one affected. It takes love and understanding from all. Life is worth fighting for! No one knows what the future holds. Only God knows how long someone will live. When cancer is a part of your life, you know you have an enemy and have a chance to fight that foe. My sincere advice is to enjoy all good things, big and small. Appreciate those people and things that surround you every day.

Have you noticed recently how good the air smells after the rain? How beautiful the sunset is? How precious your children or grandchildren are (even when they are destroying your furniture)? When did you last tell your spouse or significant other you love her or him? I continually remind myself to tell Marty that I love her each and every day and to do so with meaning.

An additional and important intent is to share my challenging pilgrimage with others, particularly my family and most importantly my grandchildren. They have been loving, generous of spirit, and a motivation for me to try to beat the cancer into submission. Recognizing the power of family and relationships, my goal is to prove—or at least strongly advance the conviction—that for all of us there will be a much better day.

Throughout my life in good times and bad, people around me have woven a tapestry to hold me up. Hopefully this story will not only help my family and friends as I share my journey with them but also become part of their fabric and the fabric of others who may read about it. My intention is to provide a gift to each of you while I acknowledge His amazing grace. I wish you love and good health!

Acknowledgments and Gratitude

Gratitude unlocks the fullness of life. It turns what we have into enough, and more. It turns denial into acceptance, chaos to order, confusion to clarity. It can turn a meal into a feast, a house into a home, a stranger into a friend. Gratitude makes sense of our past, brings peace for today, and creates a vision for tomorrow.

—Melody Beattie
Author of *Codependent No More*

For me, the most powerful aspect of the word *gratitude* is its kinship with grace. I believe that when we give thanks—whether for the best of times or the speck of light in the distance during the worst of times—we are inviting grace into our lives.

I look around me and across this land, and I raise my eyes heavenward. I appraise my existence, and my heart is always filled with gratitude—not only for those things that have brought joy but for the challenges that have given me the gift of perseverance and taught me valuable lessons, even when those lessons were hard to take.

I can think of a million reasons to acknowledge the people in my life, the ones who make my day bearable when the going gets tough, the ones who make me smile, the ones who lighten my work and life loads, the ones who quietly exist in my life, the ones who left footprints in years past, the ones who touched my life in many small ways that I sometimes do not realize until much later.

Recently I read this anonymous reminder: "When an author writes a book, she writes an acknowledgments section where she pays homage to and says thanks for all the people who helped along the way." This gratitude is long overdue. There are a few people I can think of who have impacted me so deeply that words alone cannot express my gratitude.

> We are like dwarfs sitting on the shoulders of giants.
> We see more, and things that are more distant, than
> they did, not because our sight is superior or because
> we are taller than they, but because they raise us
> up, and by their great stature add to ours.
>
> —John of Salisbury
> Twelfth-century theologian and author

In writing this book, I am indebted not only to the many talented and caring people who have helped me on this journey with cancer in one way or another but also the following institutions and individuals:

To Taylor University and our class of 1960 Golden Anniversary Reunion Committee with Nelson Rediger and Delilah Earls for opening up their arms and hearts to welcome me home.

To Dennis Hensley for his incredible talent and professionalism in editing the manuscript.

To my cadre of supportive friends at the South Bay Spectrum, particularly Rory, Lonnie, Steve, Clark, Mike, Richard, Cheryl, and Merrill, who have shown in different ways the goodness of human love by which we are enabled to live together in peace and joy and who have been and continue to be very caring, supportive, and uplifting to my spirits by their understanding, support, and compassion.

To my Tuesday Night Cancer Support Community Participation Group, which is led by Dr. Christine Winkler, with whom the sharing of experiences, hopes, fears, dreams, and everything in between became a source of shared strength and support as we've talked about our individual journeys. These people and others in the Participation Group have over the years come to be an extended family, my brothers and sisters who supported me throughout this journey.

To Dr. Lee Kissel, my primary care physician, who continues to be an integral component of my health-care team and one who has been extremely insightful and helpful as doctor and friend.

To my dermatologist, Dr. Jamie MacDougall, who with the exception of one time when he has said I needed a biopsy has always been right on target and has been instrumental in saving my life.

To my urologist, Dr. Gene Naftulin, not only for his diagnostic and medical skills but also for his compassion, understanding, and support for a patient dealing with cancer.

To the medical staff of the University of Southern California's Norris Comprehensive Cancer Center, in particular Dr. Jeff Webber and Dr. Howard Silberman, for their oncological and surgical expertise and meaningful support.

To Dr. Robert Hovenstine and the Torrance Memorial Medical Center's Department of Radiation Oncology staff for their gold standard of compassionate service and performance in treating patients such as myself.

To all the staff of The Angeles Clinic and Research Institute, the people behind the scenes. Without them, there would be a large lack of excellence in patient care. Although some people often say these things without feeling or meaning, know that this is truly how Marty and I feel.

To The Angeles Clinic and Research Institute infusion nurses—my angels—and in particular Secela, who was and remained my Angel throughout the experimental clinical trials.

To Dr. Leland Foshag, my oncological surgeon, who was always a consummate professional with a sense of humor and skillful eye-hand coordination.

To Dr. Steven O'Day for his relentless and ongoing search for the treatment and cure of melanoma. There is nothing less than heartfelt gratitude for the quality of care, guidance, information, and support provided during your tenure in my ongoing journey with cancer.

To Dr. Omid Habib, my superb oncologist and friend, with profound gratitude for providing ongoing hope and compassion while analyzing, planning, initiating, and evaluating my care. His research and professionalism as well as personal integrity have been outstanding. Words of expression and gratitude will never be enough. Rest assured you have indelibly touched our lives.

To Lonnie Murphy, not only a fellow gym rat and dear friend but also one for whom no words can express, no act of gratitude can relay, no gift can represent what his support and encouragement have meant to me.

To Irv Kodiver, a dear friend who was always there for me and with whom I've shared a male-bonding experience unlike any other in my lifetime. His unfailing friendship has been one of the rewards of having cancer.

To Kathy and Bob Blume for encouraging me along the way as well as providing support for my spirits when needed.

To Barb and Charlie Ford for their years of friendship, support, and sharing their home and their lives as well as their continuing sharing of their family.

To Jan and George Glass for reaching out and drawing me into their lives; offering support, compassion, and feedback; and reminding me of what a life well-lived is all about.

To Mary and Sam Delcamp, I acknowledge with deep gratitude their mental, emotional, and spiritual support in my life.

To Jean Taber for her life and her sharing insights into the challenges and opportunities associated with cancer, and for sharing her husband Vinnie with us. Her strength of character, spiritual acumen, and her ongoing friendship have provided comfort and inspiration.

To the very best dentist and person in the wide, wide world and beyond, Dr. Marlene Schultz. Throughout my journey she has been one of the most caring, compassionate, and supportive friends in my corner. She has helped me in the writing of this book with criticism and support, with insight and sound judgment, and with great generosity in giving of her time.

To my family, you who bring much joy, challenge, fulfillment, and meaning to my life. You have been a constant source of support and encouragement, and you reinforce the wisdom of the ages that family is what life is all about.

To Michelle, our precious daughter, who so generously gave of her artistic talents and abilities, and her time, support, and love.

To Max, a grandson who was with me from the start and who inspires me and has lifted my spirits each and every day.

To David Jr. and his gracious and caring wife, Nichole, for moving, helping, caring, and being special in many ways.

To Evie and Adam, our only granddaughter and her brother, who are bundles of energy and enthusiasm and are so utterly precious.

And of course to Marty, for her love, constancy, care, and attention and for her holding my hand through every step of the way—through the diagnosis, multiple medical interventions, and healing—and for holding onto the hope and vision that healing and beating the cancer was possible.

My deepest gratitude to God for His gift to me—the gift of life—for the unlimited blessings and abundance in my life!

Homage to Life

Life's a voyage that's homeward bound.

—Herman Melville
American novelist, short story writer, essayist, and poet

This manuscript started out as a chronicle of reflections on my journey with cancer that I would share with my family and a few friends who had stood by me throughout the process. It became a book when I was encouraged to tell what had occurred from the beginning to the present. They felt that my story would convey a message of hope, determination, and risk-taking. Some used terms such as *survivor*, while others defined me as a walking miracle. Understand that all of me—body, mind, and spirit—is a gift I have received.

Cancer is a progression, not a destination. It can become a powerful teacher. Cancer can teach us to take seriously the purpose for which we live. It has educated me about the power of love and friendship and revived an exhausted spirit. I found that cancer affects everyone in the family. For those without family, it can be a frightening and lonely journey.

I have successfully recovered from more than ten significant surgeries and several relatively minor ones, completed a schedule of more than forty-five sessions of Intensive Modulated

Radiation Therapy (IMRT), and undergone two phase-one experimental clinical trials, of which one was completed and the other cut short because of my body's failure to be responsive, and I will continue to be on special prescribed medications indefinitely. I found myself in extremely unpleasant situations that caused great suffering and unhappiness, a situation that I wouldn't wish for anyone. I have experienced discomfort and disruption of my life, but I have discovered that I have the strength to overcome adversity.

Through it all so far I have learned a lot about myself and my true character while I have persevered through doubts. I feel I have grown in wisdom. Character, a wise person once said, is what we do when no one is looking. It is not the same as reputation—what other people think of us. It is not the same as success or achievement. Character is who we are. Although we often hear of lapses of character, describing its absence does not tell the whole story. What I either reinforced or learned anew became evident to me in multiple ways.

Character and its attributes became very real to me, up close and personal. I was reminded of a 1962 book whose title alone, *Perceiving, Behaving, Becoming*, has relevance today. Whether I focused on *courage, discipline, vision,* or *endurance* in my daily life or included *compassion* and *self-sacrifice* in my behavior, all of these qualities of character have stood the test of time and became integral parts of who I am as a person. My own character has grown stronger as a result of this journey.

My faith is and has been strong. I recognize that some critics of faith have argued that faith is opposed to reason. In contrast, advocates of faith argue that the proper domain of faith concerns questions that cannot be settled by evidence. My faith is an attitude, conviction, and behavior based on a relationship with God. It is not static but grows in strength and depth as I continue to nourish that relationship with our Creator. My faith has been renewed and reinvigorated through my cancer experience.

I have had wonderful cancer care. At each stage of my journey I have met highly skilled, efficient, and compassionate caregivers. I remain vigilant about my follow-up care, including a tightly monitored schedule that involves blood draws, magnetic resonance imaging (MRI), CT and PET scans, urological examinations (for prostate cancer), and ongoing dermatology reviews.

I was determined, committed, and hopeful that my partnership with and trust in my oncologists and others on my medical team would enable me to have the quality of life and time to experience my grandchildren growing up. All those on the medical team have become more than friends. Each is now an integral part of my family.

I prepared and sustained my body through an exercise program and the best diet I could maintain. Even now sticking to my commitments about diet and exercise gives me a sense of control. I also believe firmly in the power of positive thinking to affect wellness. I was made stronger by the strength of my faith as well as by the many individuals in my community of friends, family, and prayer warriors. People I don't even know have invested in me.

At some point during my recovery I found myself appreciating everything around me. When it rained, I noticed the dew on the grass and the raindrops falling on leaves with more clarity. I recognized not only the power of the ocean but its renewal and rejuvenation as I walked along the beach. I felt gratitude for having Max, our grandson, leading me on a walk to exercise or holding my hand when I faltered. The laughter and enthralling exuberance of our granddaughter Evie and her younger brother, Adam, filled my heart with joy. I have tried to make each moment with my wife, Marty, our son, David Jr., his wife, Nichole, and our daughter, Michelle, meaningful. This continues to bring joy to my soul, which in turn brings health to my body.

The songwriter and singer John Mellencamp reminds me of a truism when he sings, "Life is short, even in its longest days." No one is promised tomorrow on earth with or without cancer. But we can live today.

Samuel Golter, former executive director of the City of Hope National Medical Center, drew my attention when he was quoted as saying, "There is no profit in curing the body, if, in the process, we destroy the soul." It is now the City of Hope's credo. For me the word *soul* can refer to both the immaterial and material aspects of being human.

A famous quote on the subject of the spirit and soul is attributed to Pierre Teilhard de Chardin (1881–1955), the French philosopher and Jesuit priest, "We are not human beings having a spiritual experience. We are spiritual beings having a human experience." The soul and the spirit are the two primary immaterial aspects that Scripture ascribes to humanity. The word *spirit* refers only to the immaterial facet of humanity. Human beings have a spirit, but we are not spirits. The spirit is the element in humanity that gives us the ability to have an intimate relationship with God. The word *soul* can refer to both the immaterial and material aspects of humanity. Unlike human beings *having* a spirit, human beings *are* souls. In its most basic sense, the word *soul* means *life*. Human beings *are* souls. The soul is the essence of humanity's being. It is who we are. The spirit is the aspect of humanity that connects with God.

Hope, faith, love, and a strong will to live offer no promise of immortality, only proof of our uniqueness as human beings and the opportunity to experience full growth even under the grimmest circumstances. The clock provides only a technical measurement of how long we live. Far more real than the ticking of time is the way we open up the minutes and infuse them with meaning. The ultimate tragedy is to die without discovering the possibilities of full growth. The approach of death need not lead to denial of that growth.

Some common growth outcomes that I share with others who are cancer and trauma survivors include a deepened appreciation for life, an enhanced relationship with others, an appreciation for personal strength and endurance, a realization that *each day really is a gift*, a deepened spiritual development, and insight into the love of the adventure we call life.

Three lessons have been especially important for me in my cancer treatment.

First I know not to expect smooth paths on any journey. Life presents events that I may not seek, anticipate, or want. Though I do not have a choice in these, I do have some choice in what I do about them, not necessarily how to *fix* them but how to *face* them. And I can smooth the path with preventive measures, such as exercising, watching my diet and weight, etc.

Secondly I know through experience that there are few safe or sure shortcuts. If I do some things only partially or occasionally or if I alter or forget other things, I might save myself time or inconvenience, but I also may bring risk or harm. Then I will be the one who pays the highest cost.

Thirdly there are few absolute guarantees. Even if I try my hardest, do my best, and care the most, I may not necessarily see the happy ending I hope for or believe I deserve. All I can do is all I can do, and I just hope it works out well.

These lessons express what I can do and what I feel I should do.

Life is worth fighting for! No one knows what the future holds. Only God knows how long someone will live. (And that is a *good* thing.)

Before my wife, Marty, had her stroke and I was diagnosed with cancer, our identities were very attached to our careers. Yet the sweetness of life is elsewhere. That is the lesson I have learned through our challenges. It is the journey we are all on, the journey called life.

The Power of Diagnosis and Treatment

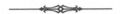

If you don't think every day is a good day, just try missing one.
—Robert Cavett
Author

From junior high school through my undergraduate years I was fortunate to be heavily engaged in sports. Coaches and teammates helped me understand the game of life. I believe that what occurs on the playing field, in gyms during practice, and in competition serves to strengthen a person's foundation for life. My athletic training helped immensely as I faced one of the biggest battles one can experience, facing cancer and being the victor.

In this chapter, I include a number of medical terms and definitions that someone interested in cancer and cancer treatment will inevitably encounter. For someone who is going through cancer therapy, these terms become a regular part of his or her vocabulary.

Another *a priori* point is that the most significant part of preventive health care is maintaining good health habits. These include

- avoiding alcohol use or using it in moderation;
- avoiding smoking and drug abuse;

- controlling diseases and disorders, such as high blood pressure, diabetes, or high levels of cholesterol in the blood;
- controlling weight;
- getting daily exercise; and
- getting proper nutrition.

Further, I would be remiss if I didn't point out that quality cancer care depends upon a team of dedicated people. The coordinated work of a team of professionals is required to provide the highest quality of care to people with cancer. When you see an oncologist (a doctor who specializes in cancer-related care), the impact of his or her dedication, compassion, and experience may be easy to recognize. However, many other people—some visible, others invisible—are working hard to provide the care needed. Of course, the most important team members are the patients and their loved ones. In the case of cancer (or any life-threatening illness), the patients are the people who take the first and most important step of getting to a doctor and undergoing intervention without delay.

How Is Cancer Diagnosed?

The earlier cancer is diagnosed and treated, the better the chance of it being cured. Most cases of cancer are detected and diagnosed after a tumor can be felt or when other symptoms have developed. Regular professional and self-examinations are encouraged for the earliest possible detection. In 2010, according to the American Cancer Society (ACS), 1.4 million Americans learned they had cancer, and many of these cases were identified through routine screenings.

In my case, I have a history of hitting my head on things, including the low ceiling in my garage. One time I ended up with a scab that was not healing on the top of my head. My very astute and caring wife looked at my scab and said she was making an appointment for me. It was then that Dr. Jamie MacDougall, a dermatologist, entered my life.

Dr. MacDougall gave me a thorough examination, including a biopsy. A couple of days later on April Fools' Day in 1997, he asked for me to come to the office. "Dave, the biopsy results came back. You have melanoma," he said.

I would be negligent if I didn't recognize that not only with his original diagnosis in 1997 but subsequently in 2002 and most crucially in 2005, Dr. MacDougall provided outstanding detection and analysis and said the magic words, "Dave, we need to have a biopsy." I came to recognize since then that his batting average with me was and has been close to 1,000 percent. Every time Dr. MacDougall did a biopsy, the results were the same. Melanoma seems to keep on giving, as it not only appeared but also progressively advanced even with appropriate intervention, including surgical removal. Dr. MacDougal literally saved my life.

Cancer Support

Supportive care from medical professionals accompanies cancer treatment from the time of diagnosis until patients are cured or expire. The goal of the cancer-care teams is to help patients with emotional and physical needs before, during, and after care. Hospice is the care for patients when they are nearing the end of their lives and assures that everything possible is done to maintain their comfort.

It should be noted here that more recently palliative care has become an integral component of one's journey with cancer. Sometimes, however, it is considered the same as hospice care. It is not. Palliative care is defined as "relieving or soothing the symptoms of a disease or disorder." Many people mistakenly believe this means you receive palliative care only when you can't be cured. Actually palliative medicine can be provided by one doctor while other doctors work with you to try to cure your illness. Palliative care is for people of any age and at any stage in an illness, whether that illness is curable, chronic, or life-threatening. In fact, palliative care may actually help you recover from your illness by relieving symptoms, such as pain, anxiety, or loss of appetite, as you undergo sometimes difficult medical treatments or procedures, such as surgery or chemotherapy. Hospice care, which is care at the end of life, always includes palliative care. But you may receive palliative care at any stage of a disease. The goal is to make you comfortable and to improve your quality of life.

Obviously I have not expired, probably because I have been the recipient of what many consider to be the gold standard of health care. I have received dedicated, compassionate, and experienced care from people who not only took care of my medical needs but also substantively contributed to fulfilling my physical, emotional, and spiritual needs. I consider myself fortunate and blessed in this regard.

What Is Cancer?

Dr. Bernie Siegel wrote in *Love, Medicine and Miracles* that 10 to 15 percent of patients want to know everything about their disease and want to become experts regarding their kind of cancer. Bernie, as Dr. Siegel likes to be referred to, also emphasizes the importance of trust in your doctor and what he or she says to you and how he or she says it. I took it upon myself to learn more about cancer, the options available in my case, and the ongoing research. In the process, I learned a great deal about my beliefs as well as myself.

Cancer is characterized by out-of-control cell growth and is classified by the type of cell initially affected. Cancer harms the body when damaged cells divide uncontrollably and interfere with body function or systems.

Angiogenesis is a normal and vital process in growth, development, and wound healing. When out of control, it is a major factor in transforming dormant tumors into a malignant (cancer) stage. Cancer cells usually use the blood and/or lymph systems to spread throughout the body. This process is called metastasis.

Apoptosis is a normal function of cells in which there is a programmed cell death, which is useful in eliminating unhealthy cells (for instance, in wound healing). When this process isn't functioning properly and apoptosis works too well or not well enough, various types of cancer are the result.

Carcinogens

There are cancers related to a cell's gene mutations (alterations) when damage has occurred to DNA or deoxyribonucleic acid (the hereditary material in humans and almost all other organisms), leading to uncontrollable cell growth. Nearly every cell in a person's body has the same DNA. Carcinogens are substances that have been directly linked to damaging DNA. They include tobacco products, asbestos, and ultraviolet radiation from the sun.

As people age, toxins and carcinogens may accumulate, which may cause DNA mutations (cell transformations). Thus, age is a risk factor. Furthermore, over time the exposure to viruses or a variety of conditions may suppress or weaken the immune system (for example, HIV, hepatitis, etc.), increasing the chance of developing cancer.

Genetic Considerations

Various genetic predispositions for cancer can be inherited. It is possible to be born with genetic mutations or a genetic fault that can make developing cancer more likely. In my chapter on nutrition, I include suggestions for foods that are conducive to maximizing health potential regardless of the other factors over which there may be no control.

What Are the Symptoms of Cancer?

Cancer symptoms vary from being nonexistent to being palpable to altering a mental or bodily function because of the cancer growth. Many cancers are found by patients during self-examination. Often oral and skin cancers are found during a routine examination by a patient's dentist or dermatologist. These lesions (any abnormal tissue found on or in an organism usually damaged by disease or trauma) may be of all colors, shapes, and sizes. If cancer spreads (metastasizes), the symptoms vary according to the extent, location, and type of cancer present.

How Is Cancer Treated?

Cancer treatment depends on the type of cancer; the stage of the cancer (how much it has spread); and the age, health status, and additional individual patient characteristics. Patients often receive a combination of therapies and palliative care. As indicated earlier, palliative care (pronounced pal-lee-uh-tiv) is specialized medical care for people with serious illnesses. It is focused on providing patients with relief from the symptoms, pain, and stress of a serious illness, whatever the prognosis. The

11

goal is to improve quality of life for both the patient and the family.

Remission is the term used when cancer is no longer detected. After a five-year period of remission a patient in many cases is considered cured. For some cancers there is no cure per se, and yet through various kinds of intervention a relapse is either prevented or the time between the no-evidence-of-disease (NED) and the relapse period is extended.

Treatments usually fall into one of the following categories:

- *Surgery*: If cancer has not metastasized, it is possible to cure a patient completely by surgically removing the cancer from the body.
- *Radiation*: Radiation treatment destroys cancer by focusing high-energy rays on the cancer cells. Radiotherapy is used as a stand-alone treatment to shrink a tumor or destroy cancer cells, and it is also used in combination with other cancer treatments.
- *Chemotherapy*: Chemotherapy utilizes chemicals that interfere with the cell-division process, damaging proteins or DNA. Chemotherapy is generally used to treat cancer that has spread because the medicines travel throughout the body. Combination therapies often include multiple types of chemotherapy with other treatment options.
- *Immunotherapy*: Immunotherapy is an attempt to get the body's immune system to fight the tumor. Local immunotherapy injects an agent into an affected area. Systemic immunotherapy treats the whole body by administering an agent that can shrink tumors.
- *Hormone therapy*: Several cancers have been linked to hormones, most notably breast and prostate cancer. Hormone therapy is designed to alter hormone production

in the body so that cancer cells stop growing or are killed completely.

- *Gene therapy*: The goal of gene therapy is to replace damaged genes with ones that work to address a root cause of cancer—damage to DNA. The most common mutation or broken gene in melanoma is the *BRAF* (V600E) gene, which has mutated in about 50 percent of melanomas.

In all, I have undergone fifteen surgical procedures, forty-seven days of radiation for prostate cancer, two phase-one clinical trials, chemotherapy (including approved and experimental "chemo cocktails"), and experimental immunotherapy. I also participated in a genetic research study, and I have been tested for the BRAF gene mutation. The only cancer therapy I have not received is hormone therapy.

Action for Cancer Prevention

I spent much of my childhood around Boston and in New Hampshire on farms. The sun wasn't as much a part of the environment as it is in California, where I live now. I always enjoyed the outdoors and loved the sun. I wanted to be bronze like so many of my friends. (It never happened for me.) I went to college in Indiana and played several intercollegiate sports. When I played baseball in college our spring break often had us playing teams in the South, particularly Florida, to compete against other colleges.

On one swing through the South I got so burned from the sun that I missed several games of pitching because I was so uncomfortable and could hardly move. After all, being young, I thought myself invincible. Advertisements reinforced the idea of getting a bronze tan as desirable! I did not ever get a bronze tan, only nasty sunburns at times. What I got later in life was not only advanced but also metastasized melanoma. One of the reasons why I am telling my story is hopefully to persuade readers to avoid the mistakes and misguided actions that were a part of my life.

Though there is no magic formula for avoiding cancer completely, there are steps one can take to improve one's odds. Many doctors and the National Cancer Institute recommend that individuals discuss cancer screening with their family physician. Screening techniques and frequency should be tailored to the patient's risk factors, including family history.

In my case, I had no family history to investigate. I was adopted shortly after birth. After more than thirty years of attempting to acquire my adoption information, I was successful, although the information proved insufficient. My adoptive parents, being deceased, were not able to shed any light on the situation.

In general, the ACS recommends the following screenings for most adults: *Breast Cancer.* Yearly screening mammograms for women beginning at age forty, clinical breast exams at least every three years for women in their twenties and thirties, and yearly for women forty and over. Monthly self-examinations in addition to professional examinations are also considered routine screenings.

- *Cervical Cancer.* Annual pap tests for all women, beginning no later than age twenty.
- *Prostate Cancer.* Beginning at age fifty, men should discuss obtaining a PSA test with their physician.
- *Colorectal Cancer.* Beginning at age fifty, both women and men should undergo screenings. Several types of screenings are available. Individuals should discuss options with their physicians.
- *Skin Cancer.* Skin examinations, both self-exams and those conducted by a physician, for men and women every three

years between ages twenty and forty and every year for anyone age forty and older.

For individuals with a significant family history of cancer (inherited syndrome), many hospitals and clinics offer genetic testing and counseling programs. I am a part of a national genetic research study intended to help researchers advance targeted treatments for cancer with similar characteristics to mine. The BRAF test (a specific test for tissue pathology regarding melanoma) has been performed to determine if I had a gene mutation, which is common in many patients with melanoma. I tested negative for this mutation.

Second Opinion

My best advice is to get a second opinion by a specialist if cancer is found or when symptoms persist and the diagnosis is not definitive. Before one begins treatment, a patient is wise to investigate by contacting several different doctors about all of the treatment options, their side effects, and the expected results. Until a patient has confidence that the treatment planned is the best option and the patient has a good relationship with the treating professionals, it is prudent to investigate by way of consultation(s) and reading about the specific cancer via the Internet. Most doctors welcome a second opinion. Some do not. Many health insurance companies will pay for a second opinion. The short delay in starting treatment usually will not make treatment less effective.

As an aside, when I was diagnosed with prostate cancer, I sought the advice and counsel of five prostate specialists, most of whom were leaders in their field of expertise. In addition, I had discussions with forty men who, in the previous five years, had undergone various treatments (surgery, radiation, hormone therapy, and watchful waiting). I did this not only to understand my options better but also to learn if the men would go through the same intervention again, knowing now what they had experienced.

I would be derelict if I didn't draw attention to a friend of mine in her cancer journey. Her name is Patricia. After a year of misdiagnosis she'd been diagnosed as having duodenal cancer (in the beginning section of the small intestine), one of the rarest forms of cancer. After having surgery as an intervention, for the next few months she experienced considerable pain and other symptoms of illness. Several months passed, and finally she was able to convince her doctors and her health insurer provider—an HMO—that there was something wrong.

Several friends, including myself, tried to convince Patricia to obtain a second opinion sooner rather than later as the months went by without treatment. We offered to assist in the process. For reasons of her own, she stuck with the original diagnosis and treatments as well as watchful waiting. Her doctors finally used diagnostic resources that showed the cancer that had remained in her body had now migrated and metastasized to several organs, including her liver. She also had several tumors on her brain.

Radiation was the doctor's intervention of choice for the tumors on her brain. After several treatments, there was indication that the tumors had been reduced in size. There also were several areas of her body, including under her eye and on her back, where there was swelling and numbness. These were diagnosed as being cysts with no need to explore further. In fact, after the radiation treatment and with knowledge that there were other parts of her body where metastasized cancer cells had migrated and tumors existed, her doctor indicated that watchful waiting would be in order until the doctor would prescribe scans to be taken to ascertain the next kind of treatment if any.

In the meantime, Patricia had been directed to a research center for possible participation in a clinical trial. However, when she was diagnosed with brain tumors, she was told that no clinical trial was available and that she had three to six months to live. Furthermore, she was advised to move into a hospice program. All of this was told to her via telephone.

Learning this information, Patricia turned to her friends and asked for some assistance in obtaining a second opinion. Her HMO would not pay for the second opinion, so she covered the expense. The consultation occurred with a wonderful, compassionate, and caring oncologist, Dr. Melani Shaum, who leads the Gastro-Intestinal Tumor Program at The Angeles Clinic and Research Institute in Los Angeles. After she finished reviewing Patricia's history, listening to Patricia's information, reviewing medical records, and interacting with her, Dr. Shaum indicated that not only were there some conventional interventions that should be provided, but there was also a clinical trial with a current opening that seemed to be ready-made for Patricia. A quick call to one of Dr. Shaum's colleagues at the clinic, who was the lead research and primary investigator on the study—Dr. Omid Hamid—indicated that an opening would be available shortly, assuming that Patricia met the criteria for the trial.

Dr. Shaum prepared a letter indicating her evaluation of the situation and made it available to Patricia and her primary doctor. Amidst the arrangements being made for her treatment, Patricia decided for personal reasons not to take advantage of the options available to her. She died a few weeks later.

The suggestion for obtaining a second opinion cannot be made strongly enough. Often it is the difference between life and death. More often than not, it reaffirms the treatment and protocols the original or primary oncologist suggested. Whatever the case, if the patient has some questions or doubts, he or she shouldn't hesitate to get a second opinion right away!

Taking Part in Cancer Research

Because of research, people diagnosed with cancer can look forward to a better quality of life and less chance of dying from the disease. Clinical trials (research studies for which people volunteer) are designed to try to answer important questions and to find out whether new approaches are safe and effective.

These are a few of the types of studies that are ongoing by cancer care professionals:

- *Active surveillance*: Doctors are comparing having surgery or radiation right away versus choosing active surveillance.
- *Cryosurgery*: Surgeons are studying a tool that freezes and kills tissue in early cancer.
- *High-intensity focused ultrasound* (HIFU): Doctors are testing HIFU in people with early-stage cancer. The process gives off high-intensity ultrasound waves that heat up and destroy the tumors.
- *Radiation therapy*: Doctors are investigating the use of radioactive implants after external radiation and are combining radiation therapy with other treatments, such as hormone therapy.
- *Hormone therapy*: Researchers are studying different schedules of hormone therapy alone and in combination with other treatments.
- *Chemotherapy*: Researchers are testing anticancer drugs and combining them with hormone therapy.
- *Biological therapy*: Doctors are testing cancer vaccines that help the immune system kill cancer cells.

My oncologist recommended to me an experimental phase-one clinical trial. (See the note at end of the chapter.) He discussed with me the pros and cons of clinical trials. For me it was an easy decision. I had to do it.

I didn't do it to try to be a hero. I already have my heroes, and the primary hero is Marty for her inspiration, inner strength, determination, and continuing commitment in dealing with the stroke that changed her life and mine in 1996.

Although clinical trials are often misunderstood and certainly make cancer patients apprehensive, confused, and overwhelmed by the diagnosis, options, language, and consent forms, my oncologist and his medical team clearly spelled out what it all was about. I understood that the clinical trial would offer the best option for my treatment. I would be able to receive a promising new medication and treatment regimen that was not yet available. I also would be a part of a significant research study. I was not going to have a placebo but would, once my eligibility was determined in meeting the trial's criteria, also receive increased monitoring and attention from the nurses and doctors because I would be in the trial. Perhaps most importantly I would be "giving back" (an important consideration for me) by furthering medical research not only for myself but also for my children and grandchildren as well as other cancer patients. Lastly I really didn't have other options other than doing nothing. Inaction was not acceptable to me. (Remember, I was given less than three months to live. In fact, without a successful intervention, according to my oncologists, I had only a few weeks.)

I completed an eight-and-a-half-month clinical trial. Three months later because of an increase in the number and size of tumors in my spleen and micro-metastasized melanoma cells elsewhere, I was able to participate in another experimental phase-one clinical trial with drugs and treatments designed to reduce or eliminate the tumors. Though it was intended to be almost a two-year trial, after eight months my tumors had been increasing in size to a point that continuing in the trial was no longer a viable option for me. Immediately the trial was discontinued, and less than two weeks later I had a surgical intervention to remove the tumors instead. I would still do the clinical trials again for the very same reasons I did them in the first place and without any hesitation.

Clinical Trials

Clinical trials are considered the best way to test new therapies for safety, effectiveness, and possible superiority to current treatments. Patients who participate in clinical trials are among the first to receive new treatments before they are widely available. There are risks associated with clinical trials because the process involves treatments that are not fully understood. There is also a chance in a clinical trial that the particular drug given in the blind testing may be a placebo (sugar pill). The known risks, potential benefits, and side effects are always part of the full disclosure prior to a patient being made part of any clinical trial.

In my case, my melanoma occurred at the IV-C stage. (Stage-four cancers have often metastasized or spread to other organs or throughout the body.) At least three organs were involved. My oncologist at the time, Dr. Stephen O'Day, presented available options to me. They were limited because I had completed radiation for prostate cancer less than six months before. A particular regimen of chemotherapy was denied by both Medicare as well as Anthem because while some "success" had been realized in patients with other kinds of cancer, the specific chemotherapies had not been approved by the US Food and Drug Agency (FDA) for melanoma treatment.

Melanoma Overview

Melanoma is a type of skin cancer, which is the most common type of cancer in the United States today, and the incidence is on the rise. Every year more than a million Americans are diagnosed with skin cancer. In fact, 40 to 50 percent of light-skinned Americans who live to age sixty-five will have skin cancer at least once in their lives. Most people think it is caused by sun damage, whether directly from the sun or from tanning beds. Though that is true in many cases, there are other risk factors for all three forms of skin cancer. Even if a person is not a fair-skinned individual or a beach bunny, he or she might be at risk.

Basal Cell Carcinoma

The most common type of skin cancer, basal cell carcinoma, is also the most treatable, especially if found early. It originates in the basal cells found at the bottom of the epidermis (the skin's top layer). This slow-growing cancer rarely spreads to other parts of the body. It tends to appear as a skin-colored or reddish bump on the head, neck, or hands that bleeds and scabs over repeatedly.

Squamous Cell Carcinoma

The second most common type of skin cancer, squamous cell carcinoma, grows faster than basal cell carcinoma, although it is also highly treatable when detected early. It can be found in the squamous cells (just above the basal cells). It is typically found on the rim of the ear, face, lips, and mouth. Though unusual, it can also spread to other parts of the body, including the scalp, neck, hands, arms, and legs. It also tends to be skin-colored or red, and it bleeds and scabs over repeatedly.

Melanoma

The least common but most serious type of skin cancer, melanoma begins in pigment-producing cells called melanocytes, which give the skin its color. It is also called malignant melanoma because it can spread to other organs. Melanoma may begin as a change in a mole or birthmark, or it may arise as a new molelike growth. Rarely melanomas can form in parts of the body not covered by skin, such as the eyes, mouth, vagina, large intestine, or other internal organs.

Rare Skin Cancers

The least common types of skin cancers include Merkel cell carcinoma, clear cell carcinomas, and sebaceous carcinomas. These behave like melanoma but arise from other parts of the skin, such as the sensory corpuscles and oil glands.

When cancer is suspected, a physician may prescribe tests to aid in the diagnosis and treatment, such as X-rays, computer tomography, or magnetic resonance imaging. When appropriate for confirming the diagnosis, a biopsy is performed, and the tissue samples are taken for microscopic examination. Other tests are done at the physician's discretion depending on the type of cancer detected.

Staging is the term used for follow-up exams to provide specific information about the cancer that has been recognized. Cancers are usually categorized from zero to four, with the lower numbers indicating those that are the least aggressive and the least invasive and that have the greatest chance of being curable. Since microscopic examination is the only way to diagnose cancer with certainty, biopsies are almost always an initial part of cancer diagnosis. A multitude of other tests may be done after this procedure to include the type, extent, and aggressiveness of the type of cancer initially diagnosed.

Melanoma is the most serious form of skin cancer and starts from pigment-producing (color-producing) cells called melanocytes. Frequently melanoma develops from a preexisting mole. Melanoma occurs most commonly on the skin of men's backs or women's legs, but melanoma can occur anywhere on the body, even in areas where there has been no sun exposure. The median age at which people are diagnosed with melanoma is just above fifty years old. Melanoma still occurs in young adults with greater frequency than many other cancer types. Treatment of the initial melanoma lesion generally involves surgery. After surgery the doctor will evaluate whether additional therapy is necessary. The vast majority of people diagnosed with melanoma are cured by the initial surgery.

In 2010, an estimated 68,130 adults (38,870 men and 29,260 women) in the United States were diagnosed with melanoma. It was also estimated that 8,700 deaths (5,670 men and 3,030 women) from melanoma occurred.

Melanoma accounts for less than 5 percent of skin cancer cases. Melanoma is the fifth most common cancer among men and the seventh most common cancer in women. Melanoma rates are more than ten times higher in white people than black people, and they have been increasing in young white women (ages fifteen to thirty-nine) and in white adults older than sixty-five.

Research done at the University of Texas MD Anderson Cancer Center in Houston, Texas, "Cancer is a Preventable Disease that Requires Major Lifestyle Changes" in a September 2008 issue of *Pharmaceutical Research* by Bharat B. Aggarwal found that cancers are primarily an environmental disease with 90 to 95 percent of cases because of environmental factors such as lifestyle and 5 to 10 percent are directly due to heredity. Common environmental factors leading to cancer include tobacco (25 to 30 percent), diet and obesity (30 to 35 percent), infections (15 to 20 percent), radiation, stress, lack of physical activity, and environmental pollutants. The ACS estimates that nearly one third of all cancer deaths in the United States each year are related to tobacco use alone.

Metastatic melanoma is the term used when the melanoma has spread through the lymphatic system to nearby nodes or through the bloodstream to other organs. It usually cannot be cured. I have been part of a monitoring and evaluation protocol that I will be undergoing for the rest of my life in attempts to identify any changes in the location and advancement of my melanoma.

Survival Rates

Experts talk about prognosis in terms of "five-year survival rates." The five-year survival rate refers to the percentage of people who are still alive five years or longer after their cancer was discovered. These are averages. Each patient is different, and these numbers do not necessarily show what will happen to an individual. The estimated five-year survival rate for melanoma is as follows:

- 99 percent if cancer is found early and treated before it has spread
- 65 percent if the cancer has spread to nearby tissue
- 15 percent if the cancer has spread farther away, such as to the liver, brain, or bones

Cancer and the Internet

Although the Internet is perceived as a huge source of information on any subject, caution is prudent on the subject of cancer as with many others. Much misguided, out-of-date, or erroneous information on the Internet may cause unnecessary worry for the cancer patient and his or her family.

Soon after I was diagnosed in 2005 with stage-four melanoma cancer, my wife and I went to visit our son and his family, who were then living on Bainbridge Island in Washington state. We had a wonderful time visiting with my son, his wife, and our latest young grandchildren. Little conversation regarding my cancer occurred during the few days we had together, and I wasn't about to bring it up.

The morning that we were to leave, I decided to get on the Internet and do some searching for sites that would provide me with insights and testimonials of those who'd had to deal with melanoma. I found a site and proceeded to read the commentaries of people who had lost family members or friends to melanoma. I then found another site and a similar series of stories. I had had enough, and I shut down the computer.

Waiting for the rest of the family to awake, my brain worked overtime. I was determined to let no one see how frightened I was. My time on the Internet sites had led me to believe my end was near, if I was to accept what I had read. As we were leaving, I held each one longer than I normally would have done and told them that I loved them. When Marty and I got in the car and drove out of the driveway, I was holding back tears. I didn't want to let my family see me in such a state. As soon as Marty and I turned right, I pulled over and burst into tears. "That probably is the last time I am going to see them," I said to Marty.

My tears and comments startled her. She touched my arm and leaned over to me. "What's the matter?" she asked.

I told her what had happened early that morning while everyone else had been sleeping. I told her about the comments that parents, wives, husbands, brothers, sisters, and many others had posted on the Internet, and I said that they weren't good. The stories related tales about treatments, pain, chemotherapy, surgery, radiation, and emotional and physical upheavals that were so negative, full of hopelessness, and full of death that, despite my demeanor up to that point, I was scared. The end result was that I decided that I would do whatever it took to beat this cancer no matter what!

When I got home from the trip, I checked out some sites from the Mayo Clinic, the National Cancer Institute, Sloan-Kettering, Johns Hopkins, MD Anderson, the Norris Comprehensive Cancer Center, and so on. My mind was put more at ease as I armed myself with helpful and insightful information. In addition, I came to realize that my oncologist, a melanoma specialist, was one of the leading melanoma researchers in the world and was highly regarded and respected.

My point is this: Although plenty of misinformation is obtained via the Internet, it can be a source for a plethora of insightful, accurate, and informative material. Before you panic, take a look at the facts. Find out whether there's any truth to these common myths about the causes and treatments of cancer.

Summary

Learn to get in touch with silence within yourself
and know that everything in this life has a purpose.
There are no mistakes, no coincidences. All events
are blessings given to us to learn from.
—Elizabeth Kubler-Ross
Psychiatrist, author of *On Death and Dying*

Among the things I quickly had to learn and apply as I moved forward from the initial unsettling news of having cancer are the following:

- *Take your diagnosis seriously.* With the help of your health-care team, an early cancer diagnosis can lead to a cure, and a late diagnosis can often lead to interventions that will either eradicate the cancer or allow for the quality of life desired.
- *Study.* Check out sound, reliable resources in your geographical location as well as on the Internet that can provide information, advice, and insights into the challenges that await you with the diagnosis you have received.
- *Skip the guilt and anger.* Don't allow yourself to begin focusing on negative thoughts and asking, *Why me? What have I done wrong?* Rather, focus on the things that need to be done and the things you can do.
- *Keep a journal.* Jot down information and thoughts, such things as what you eat and how much, your exercise regimen, and questions you have for your doctor. Share your innermost fears and concerns with your health-care team. Keep a list of conversations with medical and insurance people (include dates, names, points discussed, and actions to be taken) and appointments.
- *Maintain informational files.* Be certain to keep a file on all of your appointments and conversations with medical and insurance personnel as well as the results of laboratory work, scans, copies of reports and electronic documents, and other pertinent information and conversations.
- *Set goals.* Keep goals short and specific. Make them short-term and long-term. Review them on a continual basis.

- *Ask for support.* Be proactive in your treatment. Seek additional opinions as needed. Don't be shy about letting family and friends know specifically how they can help, and encourage them to attend support meetings. Caregivers are an essential and integral component of your treatment and recovery program.

New interventions are often studied in a stepwise fashion, with each step representing a different phase in the clinical research process. Phase-one trials are conducted mainly to evaluate the safety of chemical or biologic agents or other types of interventions (for example, a new radiation therapy technique). They help determine the maximum dose that can be given safely (also known as the *maximum tolerated dose*) and whether an intervention causes harmful side effects. Phase-one trials enroll small numbers of people (usually twenty to forty) who have advanced cancer that cannot be treated effectively with standard (usual) treatments or for which no standard treatment exists. Although evaluating the effectiveness of interventions is not a primary goal of these trials, doctors do look for evidence that the interventions might be useful as treatments.

Power of Knowledge

When cancer strikes an individual, it strikes the whole family. Fear, turmoil and loss of control are felt by all. The patient and his or her loved ones need the information and program to help empower them so that they can face the many challenges they will deal with during their cancer.

—Susan Molloy Hubbard
Former special assistant for communication,
Office of the director at the National Cancer Institute

Cancer was a disease that only happened to other people. I never thought I would get any type of cancer. Not me. No way. Not ever.

At the time when I was diagnosed with stage-four cancer, I had my sights focused on my recent retirement, travel, and time with my wife, family, and friends. I was determined to advance into the golden years and live my normal life.

The term *cancer* includes at least a hundred different types of diseases that can develop in or on any part of the body. Being diagnosed with cancer is bad enough, but not knowing what to do about it is even worse. Education about cancer is extremely important for everyone touched by this disease.

I had the need to be armed with all the information I could possibly get my hands on. I read everything I could about my type of cancer. I talked to survivors and scrutinized cancer websites.

My body has been through a lot since then. There have been surgeries, scans, chemo, and more. I had planned for my life, not for this interruption.

As devastating as a major life event can be, whether it is cancer or some other illness or event, it is this knowing from talking with friends and medical professionals and the subsequent recovery and survival that led me to believe that it—in this case, cancer—could lead me to a richer, healthier life.

In my ongoing recovery I decided to write a book, partially to convey the lessons learned concerning awareness about cancer and melanoma in particular, to make suggestions as to what has been important to me in my interaction with cancer care professionals, and to give back to all those who have helped me along this process. I have had the privilege to get to know others who have been the wounded and the survivors of the various types of cancer.

Coping with Cancer

I have been through physical and psychological challenges that battered my pride and self-esteem. At first I thought I was at the mercy of the health-care professionals. I like to be in control all of the time, and I felt completely without control when I was diagnosed with cancer. Learning about my condition helped me cope and feel more in charge of my destiny.

When told that they have cancer, many individuals may feel they have lost control of their lives. They often are overwhelmed by all the decisions they have to make. Such feelings are normal, but they need not keep the individual from taking action. You can learn about your type of cancer at your own pace. Learning and knowing what to expect are other ways to feel and be in control. It may also help to keep as normal a routine as possible. However, be patient. Coping with cancer requires an outlet for emotion, a fighting spirit, and support.

Perhaps the most illustrative story of my lack of control occurred shortly after my dermatologist informed me of my stage-four melanoma. Efforts had been unsuccessful to reach one of the leading melanoma specialists in the world, Dr. Jeff Weber, who was then at the University of Southern California Norris Comprehensive Cancer Center and Hospital. Marty and I were dining with friends of ours, George and Lisa Dutra, at their home in Prescott, Arizona. We stayed there for a couple of days to "get away from it all." As dinner was about to be served, I received a telephone call on my cell phone, letting me know that Dr. Weber's secretary would be calling me momentarily to set up an appointment. I thanked my dermatologist for his help, and the person on the other end of the phone hung up. With the cell phone still firmly placed next to my ear, I started to poke around in my pocket.

Lisa looked at me with an inquisitive smirk on her face and asked, "What are you looking for?"

"I can't find my phone. Where is my cell phone?" I was raising my voice, anxious that I would not be able to receive the anticipated important phone call.

With a smile on her face, Lisa kindly looked at me and said very calmly, "Dave, it is sticking to your ear."

The American Association of Clinical Oncology suggests that cancer patients consider taking the following steps:

- *Learn about your cancer.* Understand as much as possible about the particular type of cancer.
- *Know your options.* Discuss with your doctor treatment options for your cancer—surgery, radiation therapy,

chemotherapy, hormone therapy, active surveillance (watchful waiting), participation in a clinical trial, or not receiving treatment.

- *Understand the goals of treatment.* Treatment may be used to slow, stop, or eliminate the cancer.
- *Learn about the risks and benefits of each treatment option.* Different treatments have different risks as well as potential side effects.
- *Obtain a second opinion.* Most physicians encourage a second opinion from an oncologist or other specialist.
- *Find help managing the cost of cancer care.* Health-care teams have the resources to suggest ways to reduce and/or manage medical and associated costs, which may be high.
- *Consult helpful sources.* The American Society of Clinical Oncology (ASCO) and other cancer organizations publish guidelines and treatment decision-making materials to help the patient understand various treatment options. Discuss choices with your cancer care team.
- *Talk about your decision with people you trust.* Cancer patients frequently feel isolated initially, but a large number of people affected by this disease are willing to be supportive and share their experiences.

The Role of Statistics

Statistics cannot predict how well a treatment will work for an individual. No doctor can tell absolutely what the chances are of being cured or dying, no matter in what stage a patient might be.

Each individual and each cancer is unique. Individuals who are diagnosed with advanced stages (higher numbers) have a poorer prognosis for both cure and survival, but that does not mean that people in advanced stages will have poorer outcomes. There is no hard rule about ability to survive as it relates to cancer stages. The stage of a cancer is a description (usually using numbers one to four, with four being more progressive) of the extent to which the cancer has spread. The stage takes into account the size of a tumor, how deeply it has penetrated, whether it has invaded adjacent organs, how many lymph nodes it has metastasized to if any, and whether it has spread to distant organs.

Importance of Knowledge

I had never heard some of the simplest of medical terms. It became apparent that I needed to learn everything I could to empower myself. With cancer, knowledge can be the difference between life and death. The more that we learn, the better decisions we can make.

A well-informed patient has better capacity to evaluate the best application of resources and the best medical practices. As a word of caution, there is a lot of information on websites that may not be accurate. Don't believe everything you hear or read. Talk to a professional you trust to evaluate the accuracy of information. Testimonials and anecdotal accounts may be sincere and persuasive but might not be based on fact or have a sound medical basis.

Cancer Information

Your physician should be one of the primary sources of information. It may be helpful to request permission to tape-record discussions with your physician or to ask a friend or relative to accompany you and take notes. This will enable you to review the information thoroughly at a later time.

Most major hospitals and cancer institutions maintain up-to-date medical libraries and cancer resources for their patients. They frequently offer lectures on supportive care, individual and group support sessions, and classes on pertinent subjects.

Other sources of reliable information include the following:

- The National Library of Medicine has a free service called Medline (http://www.nlm.nih.gov/medlineplus/), where eleven million scientific studies are archived.
- The American Cancer Society at www.cancer.org has cancer information and links of interest to other cancer resources.
- For news about ongoing research, current cancer information drugs, and an online dictionary, go to the National Institute of Health's cancer research group, which is located online at www.cancer.gov. Other reputable sites worth a visit are www.oncolink.com, sponsored by the University of Pennsylvania Cancer Center, www.cancersociety.com, and the National Cancer Institute's Cancer Information Service at www.cis.nci.nih.gov.

Good Medical Care

"It's probably the most important thing in your cancer care that you believe someone has your best interests at heart," said Dr. Anna Pavlick, director of the melanoma program at the New York University Cancer Institute. "In an area where there are no right answers, you're going to get a different opinion with every doctor you see. You've got to find a doctor you feel most comfortable with, the one you most trust."

How do you decide where to go for cancer treatment? Will your chance of surviving be significantly different at one cancer center, clinic, or hospital versus another? Are some hospitals or treatment centers more successful with your type and stage of cancer than others? All of these questions begin with a conversation between the doctor and patient to determine what is best for the individual patient. Then seek information from trusted and recognized sites.

Finding a doctor and treatment facility for my cancer care was an important step toward getting the best treatment possible. Although the health-care system is complex, resources are available to guide you in finding a doctor, getting a second opinion, and choosing a treatment facility. One way to find a doctor who specializes in cancer care is to ask for a referral from your primary care physician. You may know a specialist yourself or find one through the experience of a family member, coworker, or friend.

In my case, my dermatologist, an experienced and knowledgeable person whom I trusted and whose opinion and judgment I respected, highly recommended one of the leading oncologists and melanoma specialists in the Los Angeles area, the country, and indeed the world. (People always want to believe that their doctor or specialists are world-class, but in this case, a review of the facts bore the accolades and attributes provided to me. My own research reinforced the information as well.)

Once my doctor's opinion about the diagnosis and treatment plan was reached, I chose to move forward with him and his colleagues. Other patients might want to get another doctor's advice before they begin treatment. This is known as getting a second opinion. This can be done by asking another specialist to review all of the materials related to the patient's case. A second opinion can confirm or suggest modifications to the original doctor's proposed treatment plan, provide reassurance that all options have been explored, and answer any questions the patient may have. Here again, when meeting with my medical team, I asked several pertinent questions, and all were answered with patience and knowledge.

Getting a second opinion is common, and most physicians welcome another doctor's views. In fact, your doctor may be able to recommend a specialist for this consultation. However, some people find it uncomfortable to request a second opinion. When discussing this issue with the doctor, it might be helpful to express satisfaction with your doctor's decision and care and to mention that you want the decision about treatment to be as thoroughly informed as possible. You might also wish to bring a family member, friend, or patient advocate along for support when you are asking for a second opinion. It is best to involve the original doctor in the process of getting a second opinion because the doctor will need to make your medical records (such as test results and X-rays) available to the specialist.

Choosing a treatment facility is another important consideration for getting the best medical care possible. Although you may not be able to choose which hospital treats you in an emergency, you can choose a facility for scheduled and ongoing care. If you have already found a doctor for your cancer treatment, you may need to choose a facility based on where the doctor practices. The doctor may be able to recommend a facility that provides quality care to meet your needs. Here again my decisions were made easy because my medical teams were affiliated with outstanding medical care facilities, nationally recognized, and covered by my insurance plans.

If you are a member of a health insurance plan, the choice of treatment facilities may be limited to those that participate in the insurance plan. The insurance company can provide you with a list of approved facilities. Although the costs of cancer treatment can be very high, you have the option of paying out-of-pocket if you want to use a treatment facility that is not covered by your insurance plan. If consideration is being given for paying for treatment out-of-pocket, you may wish to discuss the possible costs with your doctor beforehand. You may also want to speak with the person who does the billing for the treatment facility. In some instances, nurses and social workers can provide you with more information about coverage, eligibility, and insurance issues.

I saw Dr. Jeffrey Weber (now the director of the Donald A. Adam Comprehensive Melanoma Research Center at the H. Lee Moffitt Cancer Center and Research Institute in Tampa, Florida) at the USC Norris Comprehensive Cancer Center and Hospital and then Dr. Steven J. O'Day, Chief of Clinical Research and Director of the Melanoma Program at The Angeles Clinic and Research Institute in Santa Monica, California. I also consulted with Dr. Omid Habib, who was then associate director of both the Clinical Research and Melanoma Program at The Angeles Clinic and Research Institute.

Dr. Habib is now the director of the melanoma program and chief of immunotherapy and translational research at The Angeles Clinic and Research Institute and my primary oncologist. He has been and continues to monitor me very closely. Dr. Hamid works to ensure that patients receive access to the most up-to-date therapeutics based on molecular pathways of melanoma progression. Dr. Hamid oversees a program that ensures all types and stages of melanoma patients have opportunity to benefit from therapy.

The Power of Resources

The inequitable distribution of health-care resources in this country is generally recognized and accepted as a characteristic of American medicine. Essentially geography and financial resources determine access to health care for us.

In advance of consultation or treatment appointments, determine what you want to get out of your appointment and write your goals and ideas down to take with you. Be completely honest with the doctors about everything you put into your body—legal, prescribed, or illegal drugs.

I am reminded of the consultation with my radiation oncologist, Dr. Daniel Hovenstine. After about an hour and a half of questions and answers with him, my wife was asked to step out of the room, as he wanted to examine me more fully. After my wife left the room, he said to me, "Before you get out of your clothes, is there anything that you want to tell me that you didn't want to say in front of your wife? Sometimes patients are embarrassed to say the whole truth, or at a minimum they are embarrassed or reticent to say things in front of their spouses or significant others for any variety of reasons. I want to make sure that I have the complete picture of what you are experiencing and if there is more that can be told."

Advocacy

According to the *World English Dictionary*, advocacy is defined as "active support, especially of a cause." Being one's own advocate or having someone who can speak for you is an important asset when you are dealing with cancer. I wanted to have a level of mutual trust and respect with those who were going to pinch, probe, and analyze my body. I wanted them to share their insight and experience with me, not as a statistic but as a human being.

Personal responsibility is critical for true optimal health. Today's physicians are busy people and have great numbers of patients to care for. Patients have a responsibility to keep precise records. In order to be one's own health advocate, it is necessary to do the following:

1. *Be in tune with your body.* Keep a record of symptoms that occur. Be aware of foods or liquids that appear to cause or alter these symptoms.
2. *Do research.* Investigate the resources available.
3. *Find the right practitioner.* It is usual for cancer patients to have consultations with an oncologist who can bring together a multidisciplinary team that is critical to one's diagnosis and treatment. Feel free to seek additional opinions from professionals in the field.

Insurance

When it comes to insurance, knowledge is power. Keeping up with the paperwork from insurance carriers and health-care providers is daunting. Someone beside the patient needs to know where the pertinent information is located.

Ricki Hasou, a senior managed care analyst with the University of Texas MD Anderson Cancer Center, offers a few simple strategies to make it easier. "Know your policy, ask questions when you don't understand, and learn how to appeal a denial. And write it all down." She also adds, "Ask away. It's okay to question a charge or a denial of coverage. If you've been refused, stay polite and businesslike. Ask how you can appeal the denial." (Read the whole article in the Spring 2010 issue of *Network* at http://www.mdanderson.org/publications/network/issues/2010-spring/managed-care-issues.html.)

The nonprofit, nonpartisan Kaiser Family Foundation has an Internet site (http://www.kff.org/) that includes helpful and practical information about health insurance policies, including a printable checklist on which to record the basics of an individual plan. Knowledge about your insurance coverage really is power.

Additionally, the Affordable Care Act (ACA), implements State specific health insurance exchanges which are online price comparison websites where consumers can purchase health insurance. One can learn more about ACA and specific state health insurance exchanges by various means, including the internet site, http://obamacarefacts.com/state-health-insurance-exchange.php.

Knowledge Gained

Here in summary are selected insights gained through my experience:

- *You are the best advocate for your health.*
- *If you want or need a second opinion, get it.*
- *Copies of medical records belong to the patient.* That includes copies of radiology reports, pathology reports, surgical reports, doctor visit notes, blood test results, etc. Keep your own records and copies of every written communication.
- *Educate yourself by every available means.* Use caution, as many sources provide misinformation.
- *Get to know your pharmacist.* Ask your pharmacist about the medications and the interaction of the medications prescribed.
- *Talk to other survivors, nurses, and physician assistants.*
- *Verify the infusion medications being administered to you.*
- *Be honest and forthright with your doctor about everything.*
- *Tap into your inner resources.* Believe you will succeed in combating cancer. Consider attending support groups with people who have similar disease processes.
- *Determine how to enhance your will to live and quality of life.*
- *Set short-term and long-term goals.*

- *Seek ways to cope with or to overcome physical, emotional, and financial obstacles.* Hundreds of thousands have lived through this same experience. Communication with others has been extremely beneficial to me.

Knowledge, in truth, is the great sun in the firmament.
Life and power are scattered with all its beams.

—Daniel Webster
US senator
Secretary of state
Orator

The Power of Caregivers

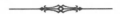

It is one of the most beautiful compensations of life, that no
man can sincerely try to help another without helping himself.
—Ralph Waldo Emerson
Philosopher, clergyman, orator

It may be a spouse, child, or friend who suffers a sudden event,
such as a stroke or accident. It might be a slower-moving, disabling
illness, such as dementia or Parkinson's disease. It oftentimes
is cancer. Whatever the case, an individual suddenly may be
changed into a caregiver who has the principal responsibility for
caring for or supporting another.

The physical and emotional strains on a caregiver are
overwhelming, and those not intimately involved in the
situation might not be aware of the scope of the burden that
is part of caregiving. In some cases, the caregiver is a young,
healthy individual. Other times an aging spouse may have the
responsibility of providing hope and healing. In my case, my wife
was my primary caregiver. As a result of a stroke several years
before, she has weakness in her arms, hands, and legs. Now our
roles were reversed.

For the caregiver shouldering the burden of the work, making
the loved one comfortable, researching treatment, interacting

with physicians, reporting news, and calming others, prayer is a blessed moment of calm in an otherwise turbulent time. Marty and I were partners in this new experience. At this time life does not go on with any sense of normalcy. Time and space are altered. Often caregivers feel alone and unprepared for this new role, as was the case with my wife.

With cancer, oftentimes the job is so overwhelming the caregiver can forget his or her own needs. A member of the cancer care team, the caregiver must often be reminded that one of the most important parts of being a good caregiver is taking care of his or her own physical, emotional, and spiritual needs first so that he or she can be the best caregiver possible.

Having been a caregiver, I can say from personal experience that there is a sincere desire to protect the one who is suffering from the compounded weight of the distress and darkness the caregiver is experiencing in dealing with the catastrophe. When one whom we love is in danger, we ourselves face darkness. The overriding question is this: How do you deal emotionally and physically as a caregiver not only while you are performing your usual tasks in the family but also while shouldering new responsibilities that are strange and unfamiliar?

There are three things that give comfort—*hope* that there will be a speedy and complete recovery, *faith* that all things are possible with the belief in God, and *love* for the one being cared for. All of this makes the unbearable bearable and turns an assault into a challenge.

As Rabbi Patricia Karlin-Neumann, the senior associate dean for religious life at Stanford University stated in her March 18, 2007, public worship sermon, "Please! Heal! Please!",

> It does, indeed, take "double vision" to see both blessing and curse, to picture opportunity amidst danger. Courage grows through hope, through the willingness to look for

unknown possibilities and to grasp them, through refusing to see only danger in darkness when its counterpart, opportunity, may be waiting in the shadows. The prayer of the caregiver, the cry of the distraught parent, the reassuring whisper of the loving spouse, can help to wrest some measure of opportunity out of danger.

Some Caregiving Roles and Responsibilities

Adjusting to a life-threatening illness is akin to finding
yourself dropped at the base of Mt. Everest and being
told to start climbing. It is a difficult task at best, but a
guide can show you the tools and techniques to make
the journey much easier. And in so doing you can
get some time to enjoy the view, now and then.

—Bob Fritz
Caregiver

The Role of the Caregiver

Unless you have a medical degree or background, chances are you don't know how to care for a cancer patient. As the husband of a stroke patient, a caregiver for a friend who had cancer, and a cancer patient over many years, I was thrust into this role. I don't have a medical degree. I had no clue. I did learn from others. I listened to doctors and nurses. I learned by doing, making mistakes, and listening to my wife during her time of need. I learned quickly, though not always easily. This was the most challenging roller-coaster ride of my life!

Even loved ones with genuine concern are challenged when they are confronted with the daunting problem of cancer. As a result, a cancer patient whose body may be undergoing treatment with the latest, most powerful drugs and technologies might still be missing out on support of his or her spiritual and emotional needs—the type of guidance that inspires hope and a sense a value in one's life even in the most challenging times.

As a caregiver, I experienced one or more of the following emotions at some time:

- *Denial*: This can't be happening to me.
- *Sadness*: Why do my loved one and I have to go through this?
- *Fear*: What does the future hold?
- *Helplessness*: I want to help my loved one, but how?
- *Isolation*: Nobody understands what we are going through.
- *Frustration*: My loved one refuses to eat. Why won't she try harder?
- *Guilt:* What right do I have to complain when my loved one is the one with cancer?
- *Being overwhelmed*: How do I sort through all of this information?
- *Anger*: Why can't things go back to normal?
- *Anxiety*: How will I take care of my loved one if the situation gets worse in the future?

These feelings are normal!

Caregiving roles can generally be broken down into three categories:

- *Live-in caregiver.* One person typically assumes the role of the primary (lead) caregiver, often for emotional, geographic, and logistical reasons. One quarter of care recipients in the United States live with their caregivers, according to the Family Caregiver Alliance.

- *Shared responsibility caregiver.* Some caregivers share supportive roles with other family members.
- *Long-distance caregiver.* In some cases, care is managed by a family member or friend who does not live near the person with cancer. A long-distance caregiver assumes the responsibility for coordinating services—often by phone or by e-mail—and arranging for local volunteers, friends, and colleagues to assist the person with cancer.

Yet I also found joy in being a caregiver. Some of the fulfilling aspects of caregiving that I found included these important attributes:

- I was able to show my wife that I was committed to providing as much needed help and support as I could.
- I helped make a difference to the quality of life and well-being of the love of my life, who was very ill.
- My caregiving helped set the tone of respect and caring for other family members regardless of their situations.

My friend Irv, a fount of insight and wisdom, provided me with the opportunity to enjoy his company as he went through his radiation and therapy treatments for prostate cancer. This became a most gratifying experience. While we spent much time going to and from his appointments, he became and continues to be a close and important friend. The experience served as an example of what life would be like if I ever had to deal with cancer. Not only did I learn my lessons well, but I also achieved a new and very close friendship!

Caring Advice for Caregivers: How Can You Help Yourself?

Most if not all focus tends to be on the patient, the one with cancer, though there may be physical and psychological hardships for the spouse or caregiver. I found several ways to cope with the challenges of being a caregiver based on my own experiences as well as those of others with whom I have been involved over the years.

- *Organize help.* Solicit help from family members, neighbors, coworkers, or professionals. Realistically there may only be one or two who have the time and/or ability to be beneficial, but you should ask. It may also be helpful to check with community agencies, religious institutions, or hospital social workers for information on volunteer and respite care programs.
- *Seek support.* Contact a support group for caregivers. Talking to others will help you explore some of the complexities of being a caregiver.
- *Become informed.* Create a list of questions for the health-care team and others who might be of assistance in coping with the situation.
- *Understand your rights.* Make yourself aware of the Family and Medical Leave Act and how it applies to family members who need time off. Some insurance companies will assign case managers to help you manage insurance concerns, clarify benefits, and suggest ways to obtain additional health-related services. The Internet is also a useful source of information.
- *Do something good for yourself.* Plan a few moments for yourself each day. A caregiver's mental and physical health

is critical in caring for another person. Diet, exercise, contact with friends, and sleep are essential.

- *Don't take it personally when the person being cared for lashes out.* Patients often are fearful, angry, frustrated, and/or depressed. Often it is difficult for a person to connect on a deep emotional level with anyone, even the people he or she loves the most. In addition, people often say hurtful things and lash out in anger. Remember that this is more often than not the illness and pain talking, not your loved one, so try not to take it personally.

The Dana Farber Cancer Institute in Boston has prepared some excellent insights into how caregivers can take care of themselves.

If you're a caregiver, you may tend to neglect your own well-being. You may not eat a balanced diet, get enough exercise, or enjoy a full night's sleep. Compared to people who are not in a caregiver role, you are more likely to experience problems such as depression, anxiety, and anger.

Watch for signs of burnout. Emotional and physical signs of caregiver stress can include:

- weight loss or gain
- trouble sleeping
- feeling depressed or overburdened
- a tendency to overreact
- feeling guilty or inadequate

Speak with a licensed social worker (LCSW or LICSW), psychiatrist, or counselor or a spiritual or religious advisor if necessary. This can help ease tension and put your experiences in perspective.

For a more complete identification of suggestions from Dana Farber Cancer Institute, go to http://www.dana-farber. org/Adult-Care/Treatment-and-Support/Patient-and-Family-Support/Support-For-Caregivers/Caring-For-Yourself.aspx.

I would add the following suggestion:

- *Attend a support group.* Seriously consider attending and participating in such groups as the Cancer Support Community. They provide a way for people to feel that they are not alone and to share important information regarding treatment, feelings, and issues.

It is a gift for the caregiver as well as the patient to be able to do the following:

- Look directly at each other and not avoid eye contact.
- Ask questions that help clarify what they're thinking and feeling.
- Make observations about what each is hearing and relating to such matters as food, pain, sleep, and other matters of concern.
- Listen. It's incredibly cathartic to be truly heard and known by someone. Each one should feel comfortable to lead the conversation and allow each other time to reveal what they are feeling.

The Cancer Support Community

Cancer changes many of the day-to-day aspects
of living, but the pursuit of happiness can go on
during the fight for recovery if you want it to.
—Harold Benjamin
Founder, The Wellness Community

I have had enthusiastic, compassionate caregivers, caretakers, and inspirational teachers. At my wife's urging I became a very reluctant participant in a Cancer Support Community (CSC). A national organization with headquarters in Washington, DC, CSC has many cancer support communities throughout the country. My local CSC is based in the South Bay area of Los Angeles.

The Wellness Community changed its name in the beginning of 2011 to the Cancer Support Community. The name change was the result of the Wellness Community's merging with Gilda's Club. The mission and focus remains the same, offering a full range of support services.

For more than twenty-five years the CSC has dedicated itself to addressing the issues of quality of life and the fight for recovery. The purpose is to serve as an integral part of the medical care for people affected by cancer. CSC's total aim is "to accurately and compassionately address all the physical, emotional, social, and practical needs of today's cancer patients, caregivers, and survivors," preparing the people impacted by cancer for wellness that hopefully will continue throughout the rest of their lives.

As indicated in *The Total Cancer Wellness Guide*, community is the most important concept of the CSC model of care that "differentiates the program from any other. People come at diagnosis, during or at the end of treatment, at recurrence, or after several years out of treatment. They all come to learn that they are not alone in their fight—whether for physical, emotional, or spiritual recovery."

There is a wedding prayer that says, "Now our joys are doubled, because the happiness of one is also the happiness of the other. Now our burdens are cut in half, since when we share them we divide the load." In our CWC program and meetings, we truly double our joys and cut our burdens in half.

Selected Research and Studies Relating to Caregivers

Studies, particularly those undertaken by the *Journal of Family Nursing*, suggest that at least 50 percent of those diagnosed with cancer will be cared for by someone in their immediate family.

According to a recent study by <u>Caring.com</u>, almost a full quarter of family caregivers care for a spouse. Forty percent of spouses who require caregiving are younger than seventy years old.

Who are the cancer caregivers?

- Eighty-two percent are female.
- Seventy-one percent are married.
- Sixty-one percent have been providing care for less than six months.
- Fifty-four percent live with the patients for whom they are caring.
- Forty-seven percent are more than fifty years old.
- Thirty-six percent reported that caregiving took more than forty hours of time per week.

Physical

- Seventy percent reported taking between one and ten medications per day.
- Sixty-two percent said their own health had suffered as a result of caregiving.
- Twenty-five percent reported having significant physical limitations of their own.

Emotional

- Eighty-five percent reported that they resented having to provide care.
- Seventy percent said their families were not working well together.
- Fifty-four percent visited friends and family less after they assumed their caregiving roles.
- Thirty-five percent said they were overwhelmed by their caregiving roles.
- Ninety-seven percent said their roles were important.
- Eighty-one percent stated that they wanted to provide care and could not live with themselves if they did not assume caregiving responsibilities

Financial

- Forty-six percent reported inadequate financial resources.
- Caregivers frequently missed as many workdays as the patients for whom they were caring, according to a survey conducted by the Fatigue Coalition (a multidisciplinary group of medical practitioners, researchers, and patient advocates).

Caregivers who participated in the University of Pennsylvania Family Caregiver Cancer Education Program reported significant increases in the degree to which they felt informed about and confident in their ability to provide care (http://www.strengthforcaring.com/manual/about-you-you-are-not-alone/cancer-caregivers/).

Cancer, Caregiving, and Hospitalization

Cancer, its treatment, and hospitalization impact the entire family. I have been fortunate that the hospital in which I had one of my major surgeries allowed my daughter to stay in the room overnight and watch over me for several days after surgery. Other family members were able to come and go at their discretion, and my wife was alleviated of some of her caregiver role—much to her and my relief, as the whole ordeal had caused her severe stress. In addition, the medical staff members—my oncologists, resident doctors, and nurses—were outstanding and provided me with a gold standard of care. Their respect, information, and welcoming approach all contributed to an environment for recovery that was greatly appreciated. In fact, my stay—and my daughter's—was so positive that my daughter wondered out loud with a smile on her face if I couldn't stay a little longer in the hospital because of the accommodations and the care we were getting!

An Inspirational Caregiver

In recent years, the concept that it takes a village to raise a child became the focus of books and commentary in the popular press. For cancer patients it is just as meaningful; however, sometimes it only takes a child. As Dr. Mehmet Oz states in the forward of *The Total Cancer Wellness Guide*, "In many ways, it takes a village—a total wellness community—to help guide the patient through the labyrinth of choices in dealing with issues ranging from dealing with the shock of initial diagnosis to creating a living legacy and a meaningful life."

One of my inspirational caregivers was a child of nine. My grandson Max has been sensitive, very special, and a source of inspiration to me. Max has been an important support in Marty's and my home and life.

In early September 2005 after I had had the melanoma surgery on the top of my head into the bone and the subsequent surgical removal of the lymph system in my neck and shoulder area, I was down in the dumps. I had bandages around my head and neck that reminded me of the characters in the 1993 movie titled *The Coneheads.*

(For the uninitiated, *The Coneheads* movie grew out of a sketch on *Saturday Night Live*, which originated in an episode aired on January 15, 1977. The Coneheads are an alien family who find themselves stranded on Earth. When questioned by Earth neighbors as to their strange behavior, they inevitably reply that they are "from Remulak, a small town in France." The Coneheads' most distinguishing feature is that the tops of their heads are shaped like large cones.)

Max, who was ever-observant, saw that for several days I had not wanted to go outside. This was unusual. The two of us often went walking or playing in a playground area after he came home from school. I was having a day filled with self-pity and was sitting in my favorite swivel rocking chair. Max came over to me and said, "Pawpaw, won't you take a walk with me?"

I said no.

Max started to take a step backward, stopped, came forward to me, and took my hand.

"C'mon, Pawpaw, you need to get up and walk with me."

I resisted once again. "No, Max, not today."

Max persisted. "Pawpaw, it will be all right. I know that you don't want to be seen the way you look, but it will be all right. If others see you walking with me, they will be very envious. In fact, they will want to know where you got that new hat on your head, and they will want to wear one too."

From the mouth of babes comes a reality check. And a child will lead them!

With that, up I went, and Max, holding tightly to my hand, took me for a walk around two blocks. We did see some people, including some children. As I shied away, Max continued to hold my hand tightly, keeping me on the straight and narrow and all the while saying proudly to all whom we passed, "This is my grandfather. He has a new style of headwear on his head. If you are interested, I know where you can get one too!"

We would continue to take our walk, and he would say the same thing to each person we passed. (Thank goodness we didn't pass many!) When we got home, he led me over to my chair and told me he would do it each day until the bandages came off. I continued our walks after the bandages came off, wearing a doo-rag for about six weeks longer to ensure I didn't contract an infection.

Personal Observations as Both a Caregiver and a Patient

Having been a caregiver for my wife, Marty, I have some knowledge of the challenges as well as the opportunities that face family members and caregivers. Having the responsibility for the health and well-being of another person changed my life.

Every year I remember January 30, 1996, as if it were occurring again. It was that day at 1:30 a.m. that Marty had a severe stroke. She spent several days in an intensive care unit (ICU) before she underwent rehabilitation and recovery in an acute rehabilitation hospital. We experienced unimagined challenges. It was a crisis.

During the period when I was with Marty 24-7 in the ICU and then in the acute rehabilitation hospital, I attempted to understand what I could do better to address what we faced.

When my wife had had her stroke, I'd called 911, and the emergency personnel had arrived within less than five minutes. The ambulance had taken her to the hospital. Our family doctor had called in the neurologist who'd saved her life.

At one point I stepped outside the ER to get some fresh air. I was frightened that the love of my life had been through all of this. She might die. I didn't want to lose her. She made me whole. How could this happen? What did I need to do? Questions and more questions raced through my mind.

I phoned our two adult children. Our daughter, Michelle, lived fairly close by, and our son, David Jr., and his family lived on Bainbridge Island near Seattle. After I hung up, I had to do something to help. I inquired what the next steps would be in her care. I held Marty's hand, stroked her head, and whispered in her ear to be strong. We could get through this. I became a caregiver, but I knew very little at that time how much there would be to do.

I arranged doctors' appointments, blood tests, CT scans, MRIs, PET scans, and other treatments. I researched treatment options, obtained prescriptions, researched other specialists, and scheduled friends to visit. Visits to various acute rehabilitation hospitals and facilities also were on my agenda. During all of them I had my son by my side, as he had taken the first plane that he could get on from Seattle to Los Angeles. I read about experimental drugs, filled out insurance paperwork, bought new pillows, and appealed countless insurance decisions. I tried to be by Marty's side through it all.

Yet despite the never-ending to-do list that could rival any CEO's daily agenda, it was never enough—never enough to do the one thing I wanted to do more than anything, specifically make the stroke disappear. In the end I had to accept the hardest item on any caregiver's to-do list. Some things were simply unachievable, and I had to learn to let them go.

As I soon came to understand from one of my Chinese friends, the Chinese word for *crisis* consists of two characters, danger and opportunity. While some linguists disagree with this interpretation, for my purposes I choose to embrace the motivational aspects of the common definition. For Marty, the danger was clear, but the opportunity for us was less apparent. We didn't yet know Marty's ultimate outcome.

When I was diagnosed with cancer and its recurrence, similar danger was present. But glimmers of light did shine brightly as we moved to higher ground in our thinking and focus. Then Marty was the caregiver.

The diagnosis of a terminal illness complicates daily existence. Anger is a common response. The patient's anger may even be directed at the caregiver, the person who most wants to be the patient's advocate.

It is not surprising that the diagnosis of a life-challenging illness creates distress. We can choose to view this crisis either as a threat to our relationship or as an opportunity to strengthen it. Kindness, patience, and love will defuse almost any power struggle. If all parties—patients and caregivers—make a commitment to adopt these qualities, the relationships will be strengthened by whatever they face on the journey with cancer. The answer to most questions for many begins with faith. Faith (spirituality) can be a compelling component in cancer care.

A Prayer for the Caregiver

Unknown and often unnoticed, you are a hero nonetheless.
For your love, sacrificial, is God at his best.
You walk by faith in the darkness of the great unknown,
And your courage, even in weakness, gives life to your beloved.

You hold shaking hands and provide the ultimate care:
Your presence, the knowing, that you are simply there.
You rise to face the giant of disease and despair;
It is your finest hour, though you may be unaware.

You are resilient, amazing, and beauty unexcelled,
You are the caregiver and you have done well!

—Bruce McIntyre
Author and inspirational speaker

The Power of Nutrition

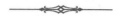

Let your foods be your medicines, and
your medicines your food.

—Hippocrates
Father of medicine

After the initial shock of the diagnosis of cancer, there are decisions
that need to be made. The treatment options may be many or few.
The cancer care team will offer choices and advice about what is
most appropriate. One topic that probably will not be discussed is
what is put into your body by way of nourishment. That was my
experience, and others have shared similar observations. Nutrition
comes in two forms—one kind for the mind and one kind for the
body. These are things over which only the patient has control at
a time when there may be a devastating feeling of loss of control.

Even small choices are important in being a participant in
care. Patients frequently feel powerless as physicians regulate
aspects of care like chemotherapy, radiation, and surgery. Studies
have shown that individuals who are active participants in their
cancer care feel better about themselves and are more positive
about the future. I took the recommendations and applied them
to my own situation. By taking charge over what was put into my
body, I became an active, involved member of the cancer team.

Nutrition is important for everyone. Many health problems can be prevented or alleviated with the proper nutritional intake. This has special meaning when cancer develops. It did for me.

There are many things one cannot control, including genetics and disease. However, proper foods make a difference in strength and mental attitude during cancer. According to the World Health Organization (WHO), a wholesome intake of food and water is important for the prevention of chronic health conditions as well, such as obesity, heart disease, diabetes, and cancer.

Adequate nutrition may become compromised during cancer therapy. In some cases, head, neck, or gastrointestinal tumors interfere with eating and/or swallowing. In other instances, the treatment itself may decrease the patient's appetite, induce nausea, or cause food aversions. Keeping your team apprised of symptoms that limit your ability to take in the necessary nutrients is essential to recovery.

Post-Surgery Experiences

It is amazing what the mind can do! In my case, after a significant surgical procedure on the top of my head lasting a little more than six hours, I found myself with my feet tied down and a pumping sensation in my legs. (Actually it was an intermittent pneumatic compression around each leg.) A picture emerged in my mind of a cow being milked by the suction cups placed over her teats. I also discovered that I was hungry after I had been under the knife for several hours and after I had fasted in preparation for the surgical procedures. I was hungry … very hungry.

I remember twisting and turning in an effort to figure out what each of the many tubes that emanated from various parts of my anatomy to unseen places were doing. Though my glasses were somewhere close by, I didn't see them, but lo and behold, there was a nice white Styrofoam cup filled with crushed ice.

Waking up after being removed from the surgical recovery room to my hospital bed and a night of panic as well as humor, I found myself restrained. (The humor was a result of one of the machines feeding me intravenously became empty and bells went off as they are prone to do. In a state of panic after waking, I reached for what I thought was the button to ring the nurse. Instead it was the button to increase the pain medication automatically and I quickly fell asleep only to repeat it several times during the night. No longer did I hear the bells going off!) I have no memory of any of this occurring since I was heavily sedated—thank goodness— but apparently I resisted quite strenuously.

In the waiting room my wonderful wife waited along with Mary, one of our dear friends who'd stayed with her through the whole surgical procedure. A nurse approached them. "May I ask what your husband does for a living?"

My wife was puzzled by the question and inquired, "Why do you ask?"

"Well," said the nurse, "your husband is very strong."

"What happened?" Marty asked.

"We normally have little difficulty with the catheter insertion," said the nurse. "However, it took six male nurses to hold your husband down so that we could get the catheter in, and even then your husband didn't cooperate!"

With a smile my wife responded, "Well, he does work out at a gym almost every day."

The nurse smiled back and said to my wife, "Tell him to keep it up but don't practice on us. We had one of the most difficult times I have ever had in my twenty years of working in the recovery room."

When I was a little more awake and somewhat lucid, I asked the nurse if she could find my glasses and give me that Styrofoam cup. My mouth was parched, and I wanted to feel something going into my mouth, throat, and beyond to curtail the hunger pangs I was feeling. At the same time I was told in no uncertain terms that I was not able to eat any solid foods and that one of the tubes entering my body was a feeding tube and that was all the nourishment I could have for a couple of days or so.

Soon I had my glasses on, and the cup of crushed ice was placed in my hand. As I raised the cup very slowly and gingerly, a small stream of liquid from the ice that had melted began cascading over my tongue. I savored the taste, the coldness, and began thinking about what I was doing.

Besides the liquid, a few pieces of the crushed ice began to enter my mouth. It was heavenly! Soon in my mind it became milk, and the small pieces of crushed ice became eggs. A little later the mixture became cereal and milk and then a small sip of juice. Soon my hunger pangs were gone, and I had a full stomach. It was amazing what my mind had been able to do.

A little later with my mouth feeling dry, I reached over, and thankfully my precious nurse had brought in another cup of crushed ice while I'd been napping. I repeated the same ritual. This time, however, the crushed ice and water that had melted became fresh orange juice, fulfilling my nutrition needs for the moment. At lunchtime the crushed ice became a bowl of soup along with my fantasized piece of bread and a banana with some additional fruit.

For my first dinner I decided in my mind's eye that a small steak, baked potato, some fresh vegetables, and a small fruit cup for dessert would satisfy my hunger and my dinner needs. Since my nurses had discovered that crushed ice was my food of choice—as if I had a choice—they kept my side tabletop filled with crushed ice. After my meal I fell asleep again with a smile on my face and happiness in my belly. Later even my fantasy of Chinese food tasted delicious.

A day or two later I was able to begin to eat more solid food, though most of it was gelatin at first, and I thought that I wanted to go back to my crushed ice. It tasted better!

The Importance of Good Nutrition

An often cited article by Ose, et. al, that appeared in the September 20, 1998, *Journal of the Norwegian Medical Association*, "The importance of nutrition for cancer patients," reinforces the fact that good nutrition is vitally important for cancer patients before, during, and after treatment.

Cancer treatment kills cancer cells, but to varying degrees it also damages healthy cells. The risk of cancer itself can be reduced by as much as 40 percent, according to the MD Anderson Cancer Center, by making healthier food choices. In fact, some foods can actually help protect against certain cancers. Eating a plant-based, healthy diet (fruits, vegetables, whole grains, and beans) in addition to being physically active is the best insurance to reduce the risk of cancer as well as other diseases, such as heart maladies and diabetes.

In the September 2001 issue of *Nutrition*, Capra et al. indicate that nutritional screening is an important aspect of overall treatment. It is important to work closely with the cancer care team to assure that the patient maintains nutritional intake, whether by regular food, dietary supplements, or external (IV) methods. Malnutrition can be avoided in most cases, even in advanced cancer.

Side effects of cancer treatment that make it difficult for patients to eat include gastrointestinal symptoms, sore and/or dry mouth, sore throat, dental problems, changes in the senses of taste and/or smell, fatigue, and psychological problems (depression and/or anxiety). The effects of cancer and cancer treatments may make it hard to eat well. Absorption of nutrients may be an additional issue, particularly when the head, neck, esophagus, stomach, and/or intestine are affected by the cancer treatment. Though I didn't experience all of the symptoms, I did have a loss of taste and smell, fatigue, and a decline in my appetite.

Surgery, chemotherapy, radiation therapy, immunotherapy, and stem cell transplant can all affect nutrition. Here are some suggestions that may help based on my experience.

Eat a regular breakfast or lunch on the day of chemotherapy. If the appointment for chemo is a late-morning or afternoon appointment, eat a snack before treatment. Avoid fried or greasy foods. In the absence of my breakfast of cereal or a protein drink on the mornings that I had my chemo treatments, I found that oatmeal in a small amount was very helpful.

Eating frequent small meals may be helpful to prevent nausea. Avoid spicy foods, red meat, and foods with strong odors. Some easy snacks that I found helpful and enjoyable are bland fruits, bland vegetables, cereal, eggs, sugar-free ice cream or sherbet, oatmeal (worked well for me), pasta with mild sauce, pretzels, skinned chicken, toast, crackers, waffles, or yogurt.

Cancer care teams also have medications to help control the nausea and vomiting, which may be a side effect after one receives chemotherapy.

It is not uncommon for food and drinks to taste different while one is receiving chemotherapy, which can reduce the desire to eat. Avoid using metal utensils for eating if a metallic taste is a problem. Use herbs and mild spices to enhance flavor if foods have an unpleasant taste.

A significant person often overlooked in the treatment of most cancers is the dental professional. I have been extremely fortunate in having access to a dentist who is also my friend. The importance of seeing your dentist immediately upon the diagnosis of cancer cannot be overstated. Ask your dentist if he or she is comfortable in working with you on the effects of the various cancer therapies that you may be undergoing. Dental schools usually have departments and experts who work with patients undergoing cancer therapies of all kinds.

Seeing your dentist several weeks *before* beginning the cancer treatments assures the best chance of avoiding oral problems that will affect your ability to consume nutrients and helps prevent pain and suffering from dental decay and/or tissue soreness during cancer treatments. Pretreatment dental care may involve complete X-rays, fluoride tray fabrication, education about oral and lip dryness, information about the use of the proper dentifrices and nonalcohol mouth rinses, restoration of any decayed teeth, and detailed oral hygiene instructions.

With the dry mouth that accompanies some cancer therapies and medications, the plaque that builds in every mouth becomes a sticky substance that can cause decay, gum problems, and mouth sores. Unfortunately when mouths are sore, it is natural to turn to sweet, feel-good, nonnutritious foods that may have a detrimental effect on the teeth and overall health.

Certain cells (phagocytic) that clean up infected areas are less active when sugars are introduced into the food intake. Stick with soft foods that do not contain sugars or sugar-free (not sugarless) baby foods when the tissues of the mouth are sensitive.

Cancer and the Way the Body Uses Food

Some tumors make chemicals that change the way the body uses what has been ingested. The body's use of protein, carbohydrates, and fat may be affected, especially by tumors of the stomach or intestines. A patient may seem to be eating enough, but the body may not be able to absorb all the nutrients from the food.

When the body does not get or cannot absorb the nutrients needed for health, it may cause *malnutrition*. Cancer patients are in danger of malnutrition because of the side effects of the treatments.

Malnutrition

According to the National Cancer Institute, about one third of all cancer deaths are related to malnutrition. If malnutrition continues, the conditions for survival are threatened, and muscle, fat, and tissue wasting (deterioration) begins.

Malnutrition occurs when the supply of nutrients and energy is inadequate to meet the body's requirements. Insufficient food intake can result in *anorexia*, a progressive condition in cancer, where the individual loses interest in food intake or can no longer pass foods through the mouth. The individual begins to lose weight, including the muscle mass, tissue, and fat necessary for healing and recovery. The Wellstar Health System defines cancer anorexia as an occurrence in both early- and late-stage cancers, resulting in considerable weight loss and weakness. This can jeopardize treatment since the compromised health and strength needed to withstand chemotherapy and/ or radiation are compromised. This can also limit treatment options. Some patients already have anorexia when they are diagnosed with cancer. Anorexia is the most common cause of malnutrition.

Cachexia is a condition that often accompanies anorexia in cancer patients, and it is difficult to correct the damage once it has taken place. It is the loss of muscle, fat, and tissues as a result of anorexia and malabsorption of nutrients. Wellstar Health System warns that without prompt intervention by stimulating the appetite, maintaining nourishment and nutrition, and controlling diarrhea and vomiting, the individual will no longer respond to treatments, and survival rates become grim. Cachexia is common in patients with tumors of the lung, pancreas, and upper gastrointestinal tract.

Cancer symptoms and side effects that affect eating and cause weight loss should be treated early. Nutrition therapy and medicine can help the patient stay at a healthy weight. Medicines may be prescribed in order to accomplish the following:

- help increase appetite
- help digest food
- help the muscles of the stomach and intestines contract (to keep food moving along)
- prevent or treat nausea and vomiting
- prevent or treat diarrhea
- prevent or treat constipation
- prevent or treat mouth problems (such as dry mouth, infection, pain, and sores)
- prevent or treat pain

Cancer and cancer treatments may affect taste, smell, appetite, and the ability to eat enough food or absorb the nutrients from food. Patients may become weak, tired, and unable to fight infections. Eating too little protein and calories is a very common problem for cancer patients.

Nutrition for the Person with Cancer during Treatment

According to the American Cancer Society, good nutrition helps cancer patients maintain energy levels and avoid significant or dangerous weight loss. It helps patients heal more quickly from surgeries, strengthens the immune system, and helps to avoid infection. In addition, input of healthy foods helps patients

David E. Leveille

endure the side effects of cancer and other treatments. To put it very simply, people just feel better with good nutrition.

The American Cancer Society indicates that nutrition is a three-part process that gives the body the nutrients it needs:

- The body intakes food and drink.
- The body breaks the food down into nutrients.
- The nutrients are used as fuel, building blocks, and for other purposes.

In order for the body to receive proper nutrition, there must be sufficient foods that contain certain nutrients.

Calories measure the energy received from food. The body needs calories to fuel all of its functions. At times extra calories may be necessary to fight infection, raise the body temperature, and rebuild damaged tissues.

Benefits of Good Nutrition

Optimal nutrition allows your body to function at its best and can provide several benefits for people living with cancer, including the following:

- supporting immune function
- preserving lean body cell mass
- rebuilding body tissue
- decreasing the risk of infection
- improving strength and increasing energy
- improving tolerance of treatment
- helping with recuperation at a faster rate following treatment
- improving quality of life

68

Proteins

Proteins supply calories to the body. The energy produced by proteins is four calories per gram. Proteins are necessary for growth, repair of body tissue, promoting of healthy immune systems, speeding recovery time, and fighting infection. Good sources of protein include lean meat, fish, poultry, dairy products, nuts, dried beans, peas, lentils, and soy foods.

Fats

Fats supply calories to the body. The energy produced by fat is nine calories per gram. The body breaks down fats and uses them to store energy, insulate body tissues, and transport some types of vitamins through the blood.

When one is considering the effects of fats on the heart and cholesterol levels, it is wise to choose unsaturated fats (monounsaturated and polyunsaturated):

- *Monounsaturated fats* are found mainly in vegetable oils like canola, olive, and peanut oils and are liquid at room temperature.
- *Polyunsaturated fats* are found mainly in vegetable oils like safflower, sunflower, corn, flaxseed, and canola oils and are the main fats found in seafood. They are liquid or soft at room temperature.
- *Polyunsaturated fatty acids*, like linoleic acid and alpha-linolenic acid, are called essential fatty acids because the body cannot make these acids. These are needed to build cells and make hormones.
- *Saturated fats* (or saturated fatty acids) are mainly found in animal sources like meat and poultry, whole or reduced-fat

---

milk, and butter. Some vegetable oils like coconut, palm kernel oil, and palm oil are saturated. Saturated fats are usually solid at room temperature.

- *Trans fatty acids* are formed when vegetable oils are processed into margarine or shortening. Sources of trans fats include snack foods and baked goods made with partially hydrogenated vegetable oil or vegetable shortening. Trans fats also are found naturally in some animal products like dairy products.

Carbohydrates

Carbohydrates supply calories to the body and are the body's major source of energy. A gram of carbohydrates produces four calories. The best sources of carbohydrates—fruits, vegetables, and whole grains—also supply needed vitamins and minerals, fiber, and phytonutrients to the body's cells. (Phytonutrients are plant compounds like carotenoids, limonoids, and phytosterols that are thought to have health-protecting qualities.)

Other sources of carbohydrates include bread, potatoes, rice, spaghetti, pasta, cereals, corn, peas, and beans. Sweets (desserts, candy, and drinks with sugar) supply carbohydrates but provide nothing in the way of vitamins, minerals, or phytonutrients and may be damaging to your health.

Whole Grains

Whole grains or foods made from whole grains contain all the essential parts and naturally occurring nutrients of the entire grain seed. Whole grains are found in some cereals, breads, flours, and crackers. *Fiber* is the part of plant foods that the body cannot digest and helps to move food waste out of the body quickly.

Water

Water and other liquids or fluids are vital to health. Dehydration occurs when there are insufficient fluids in the body, perhaps because of vomiting or diarrhea for example.

Vitamins and Minerals

Vitamins are nutrients, such as vitamins A, C, and E, that the body needs to grow and stay strong. They can be found naturally in foods. Examples are iron, calcium, potassium, and sodium. They allow the body to use the energy (calories) found in foods.

Antioxidants

Antioxidants include substances like vitamins A, C, and E, selenium, and some enzymes that absorb and attach to free radicals, preventing them from attacking normal cells.

Herbs

Herbs have been used to treat disease for hundreds of years, with mixed results. Today herbs are found in many products. Some of these are harmless, and others have very negative effects. Some may interfere with proven cancer treatments, including chemotherapy, radiation therapy, and recovery from surgery.

Safety Considerations

All things that are consumed during cancer therapy must be discussed with the cancer care team. The precautions on the packages and/or bottles do not cover all possible side effects, which can include rendering some treatments and medications ineffective. The cancer care team must be involved in the decision about any supplements to the body because instead of having a beneficial effect, the supplements may interfere with chemotherapy or radiation treatments.

Strength and Stamina

In order to maintain muscle mass, stamina, and strength to withstand cancer treatment, patients are advised to keep their baseline weight constant. To counter weight loss, the Stanford Cancer Center recommends a diet high in protein and fat that includes milk and milk products, cooked eggs, sauces and gravies, as well as butter, margarine, and oils.

Cancer Prevention Diet

The diet for cancer prevention is simple and basic and is filled with vegetables and fruit for all meals and snacks. It is important to vary fruits and vegetables and eat the brightly colored ones as much as possible, as they have the most vitamins, minerals, and antioxidants. Choose whole grains when you are selecting breads, pasta, and cereals. Eat low-fat protein and fish, which is rich in omega-3 fatty acids. Avoid refined and processed foods. Plan ahead and have the freezer, refrigerator, and pantry filled with nutritious foods. In that case, it is far more likely you will consume foods that are readily available.

Nutrition during Treatment

There may be times when you do not feel like eating. Tempt yourself with some of your favorite healthy foods to stimulate your appetite. Explore new foods that are appealing in color and nutrients.

Nutrition after Treatment

Eating lots of fruits and vegetables helps keep the immune system functioning and the body as healthy as possible. According to the suggestions in Oncology Nursing News, fill plates with three-fourths vegetables at each meal. Eat healthy, high-fiber whole grains, legumes, and nuts rich in vitamins and minerals. Solicit advice from a dietitian on what minerals and vitamins should be added to the foods consumed.

The World Cancer Research Fund's *The Second Expert Report: Food, Nutrition, Physical Activity, and the Prevention of Cancer: A Global Perspective* features eight general and two special recommendations. The ten summary recommendations are listed below. Together they comprise a blueprint that can be followed to help reduce one's risk of developing cancer.

- *Body fat*: Be as lean as possible within the normal range of body weight.
- *Physical activity*: Be physically active as part of everyday life.

- *Foods and drinks that promote weight gain*: Limit consumption of energy-dense foods. Avoid sugary drinks.
- *Plant foods*: Eat mostly foods of plant origin.
- *Animal foods*: Limit intake of red meat and avoid processed foods.
- *Alcoholic drinks*: Limit alcoholic drinks.
- *Preservation, processing, preparation*: Limit consumption of salt. Avoid moldy cereals (grains) or pulses (legumes).
- *Dietary supplements*: Aim to meet nutritional needs through diet alone.
- *Breast-feeding (special recommendations)*: It is recommended that mothers breast-feed and children be breastfed.
- *Cancer survivors (special recommendations)*: Follow the recommendations for cancer prevention.

Cancer Care: What Your Body Needs

"Nutritional needs can change depending upon the type and stage of cancer," says Sharlene Bidini, RD, CSO, a board-certified specialist in oncology nutrition at the Oakwood Center for Cancer Care in Dearborn, Michigan. "Certain cancers are considered at greater risk for nutritional complications, including colorectal, esophageal, gastric, head and neck, lung, and pancreatic cancers."

Cancer patients who have an immune system compromised by cancer treatment should be careful to avoid foods that could cause further harm like unpasteurized dairy products, raw fish and meat, and other foods that are undercooked.

Those with late-stage cancer should focus on getting in as many calories as they can with small meals or snacks every one or two hours. Stick to foods that taste best, and drink plenty of fluids to stay hydrated.

Preparation for Cancer Treatment

The diagnosis of cancer used to be a death sentence. Not so anymore. According to the National Cancer Institute, negative side effects are not predetermined. Taking control of the things that you can, such as what you eat and drink, are positive steps toward recovery. This constitutes nourishment for the mind and body. Enjoy every day. I do!

The Power of Exercise

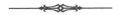

In terms of fitness and battling through cancer, exercise
helps you stay strong physically and mentally.

—Grete Waitz
Marathon champion

As I underwent my cancer experience, I was reminded once again of the importance of not only the spiritual and the mental aspects of what I was to experience but also the physical. Exercise was an integral component of my life and has continued to be a part of my daily determination to beat cancer.

In addition to knowing my body and being determined to have a normal life under the circumstances, I realized how vital exercise was to me not only in recovery but also in reducing my chance of getting the cancer back again. Though I knew that it was still in my body—metastasized melanoma is the gift that keeps on giving, but you just don't know when—I was committed to do all I could to exercise and live for years to come, God willing.

I have been in a fitness center for more than forty years. I enjoyed participating in sports at the high school and college levels and then settled into swimming, tennis, skiing, hiking, and so forth. Exercise of one sort or another has been a part of my daily regimen and prepared me well for the challenge of dealing with cancer.

I am a member of one of the Spectrum Athletic Clubs in Southern California. It offers the Cancer Wellfit Exercise Program, a ten-week mind and body fitness course designed for adult cancer survivors who have recently become deconditioned or chronically fatigued from their treatment and/or disease. The goal is to help patients build muscle mass and muscle strength, increase flexibility and endurance, and improve functional ability. Additional goals include reducing the severity of side effects, preventing unwanted weight changes, and improving energy levels and self-esteem. A final goal of the program is to assist participants in developing their own physical fitness programs so that they can continue to practice healthy lifestyles, both as parts of their recoveries and as ways of life.

When first diagnosed with cancer, I certainly didn't interrupt my exercise program. It was not because I was a zealot. Rather, I was committed to try to maintain my daily routine and regimen as much as possible. The benefits of exercise for the general population are well publicized. But what if you are a cancer patient?

Due in part to the protocols of the experimental trials that I was in, even as I was attempting to exercise and maintain my routines, I found myself becoming weaker. My waning strength reduced my weight-lifting capacity, and often I could not maintain the same level of repetitions. Nevertheless, as the cancer interventions became more intense and demanding, I was able to meet the challenges. My oncologists indicated it was because of my exercise routine as well as my determination and mind-set to meet the challenges that were part of the success of the cancer interventions.

Before I started my own multiple intervention treatments, I asked my oncologists as well as others on my medical team for

77

their thoughts. To a person, they encouraged me to maintain my exercise program and listen to my body. They all believed it would be beneficial during treatments and afterward. More importantly they believed it would contribute to the quality of life that I wanted to have.

As I mentioned earlier, people undergoing cancer treatment traditionally have been told to rest as much as possible and avoid exertion, to save all their strength to battle the dreaded disease. However, a growing number of physicians and researchers now say that people who remain physically active as best they can during treatment are more likely to beat cancer. Fortunately my medical team of oncologists, surgeons, nurses, and myriad others all encouraged me to maintain my exercise program.

Though there are many reasons for being physically active during cancer treatment, each person's exercise program should be based on what is safe, effective, and enjoyable for that person. I came to realize in no uncertain terms that my exercises should take into account the exercise program I already followed, what I could already do, and any physical problems or limits I had. In talking with my fitness guru and friend, we modified my exercise program to meet better my interests and needs.

The conventional wisdom used to be that one should just go home and rest after chemo treatment. Now that appears to be the worst thing you can do. Exercise has been shown actually to reduce fatigue during chemotherapy.

I have memories of recovering in a wonderful hospital after undergoing surgery for the removal of my spleen, part of my pancreas, and a few slices from my stomach to rid my anatomy of some melanoma cancer tumors running amok. My first exercise was to blow into an incentive spirometer (an apparatus for measuring the *volume* of *air* inspired and expired by the *lungs*) and try to make a Ping-Pong ball rise to get the lungs working.

It was extremely hard. My whole abdomen, stomach and chest hurt, but over time it did get easier.

Then the physical exercise came. At first it was just getting out of bed and walking to the door and back. That was agony followed by exhaustion.

I was encouraged then to start walking laps in the ward. Sometimes I lied, saying I'd done two laps when I did three and eventually up to about ten. The reason for my fibbing was that, on the one hand, I knew the staff didn't want me to overexert myself and have any setbacks, and on the other hand, I wanted to prove to myself that I could exceed all expectations regardless of my age and that I was capable of doing more.

I heard murmurs from other patients in the ward who thought that the nurses and staff were being very cruel by making them get up and walk the halls a few times a day. The patients were insisting that the nursing and staff members put themselves through the torture. I, on the other hand, came to enjoy walking laps and exploring the new wing of the hospital and made several excursions each day around the floor. My mind-set was that it was making me better. I was getting stronger, and it would speed my recovery as well as enable me to leave the hospital sooner. After I returned home, I walked four and then ten blocks each day before I headed to the gym. I started getting back into the swing of things on the fourth day after I had left the hospital.

I should point out that though I have incorporated three to four different approaches to my exercise regimen so that I don't get bored with the uniformity of a single regimen, almost every day I include a minimum of thirty to forty-five minutes of cardiovascular work on various machines that enable me to strengthen my heart among other parts of my body.

The Importance of Exercise

Have you ever wondered if there is *anything* that can be done to reduce stress levels, enhance abilities to perform activities of daily living, and potentially boost our immune systems? Well, there *is* something. It is called *exercise*. When engaged in safely, exercise can increase quality of life and enhance feelings of independence and self-confidence. There is no magic to it. We just need to do it!

There are ten million cancer survivors in the United States. Twenty-two percent of them are women who have had breast cancer, and 17 percent of them are men who have had prostate cancer. Exercise makes sense for most of them—to live longer, avoid other health problems, and just feel better. Heart attack patients are now routinely put on exercise plans, but workouts for cancer patients are neither prescribed by doctors nor covered by health insurance.

The standard weapons in the fight against cancer—surgery, chemotherapy, and radiation—may soon be joined by something far simpler, namely exercise. In a few years exercise will probably be prescribed regularly for cancer rehabilitation, according to Melinda Irwin, an expert on cancer and exercise at Yale University School of Medicine. Personal trainers may join oncologists, surgeons, and radiologists as members of the cancer treatment team. Exercise will become a "targeted therapy, similar to chemotherapy or hormonal therapy," Irwin said.

Any regular physical activity—the equivalent of a thirty-minute walk five times a week—will do. As Dr. Irwin says, "Don't think you have to work up a sweat or train for a marathon to benefit."

I also have a strong belief that improving one's fitness level prior to the onset of cancer treatment will improve the healing process and help maintain quality of life.

Cancer is a disease that affects people on different levels and in different ways, depending on the location of the tumor and whether the tumor is localized or metastasized. There are generalized symptoms based on the location of the tumor that must be considered when one is prescribing an exercise program—pain, shortness of breath, neural deficiencies, seizures, easy fatigue, and anemia. Additionally the goals of the exercise program will vary depending on the stage of the cancer.

Exercise offers many advantages. It fights the fatigue caused by cancer treatment, calms anxiety, and helps survivors feel better about themselves and their bodies. It also allows the organ systems to adapt positively and improve metabolic efficiency, thereby enabling more intensive cancer treatments, fewer side effects, and better sleep patterns.

Surviving cancer and making it through cancer treatment are major accomplishments. Most survivors if not all find a new priority in life—keeping cancer from returning. The latest research suggests that exercise for cancer patients may help.

What Are Some of the Benefits of Exercise as a Supplement to Cancer Treatment?

While a cancer diagnosis is often devastating, regular exercise can help minimize the effects of the disease as well as potentially increase chances for survival.

Cancer treatment is very intense. But even for people who were previously couch potatoes, exercise can be a blessing. It is a way of actively doing something to improve one's own physical and mental well-being. It provides an escape, a chance to alleviate worries and go beyond traditional medicine. It's an opportunity to do something enjoyable. It is something you can control.

Exercise will affect individuals in very different ways. Although exercise may be uncomfortable at times, the long-term benefits generally outweigh the immediate discomforts you exercise properly.

Physical Improvement

Some people with cancer, especially forms of the disease that affect the head, neck, or intestines, suffer significant body deterioration and persistent pain and discomfort. Decreased muscle mass can make performing everyday activities like getting up from an automobile seat difficult or impossible. As it did for me, even moderate exercise—including activity that takes place while you are undergoing chemotherapy or radiation—can help rebuild lean muscle, increase heart strength, and eventually make normal movements and independent living possible. The National Cancer Institute says that patients in a study who participated in daily exercise that included brisk walking experienced less fatigue than patients who did not exercise. They also developed stronger aerobic capacity and enhanced strength.

Weight Loss

Treatment for several kinds of cancer, including breast cancer, often leads to significant weight gain. Regular exercise combined with a healthy diet aids the ability to lose fat and control body weight so that eventually a healthy body mass index can be regained. Body mass index (BMI) is a number calculated with height and weight, and it is used to determine weight-related health conditions. Patients should ask their doctors what constitutes healthy BMIs for their situations.

My weight loss in a little more than eight months was forty-eight pounds. During the last two months of my second clinical trial—before it was stopped because of the growth of tumors (a 25 percent increase from the baseline size)—I lost more than twenty pounds. My white cell count was low. I was anemic because of my treatment regimen, and I was scheduled to see, among others, a nutritionist to review my eating habits as well as my food intake. Since the decision was made to have surgery before the appointment occurred, my blood work subsequently indicated that the anemia was no longer an issue, so appointments were cancelled with the nutritionist and other specialists.

Long-Term Survival

Those with cancer face a greater risk of heart problems and broken bones along with other health challenges that can threaten one's overall well-being. The threats become more significant when individuals practice sedentary lifestyles. Some studies suggest that adding exercise into a weekly list of activities may improve chances of survival from cancer, although more research is needed to prove any long-term benefits. *The New York Times* reports that colon cancer patients who exercised had a 50 percent lower rate of mortality than patients who were sedentary.

Combating the Side Effects of Cancer Treatments

From my own experience, many cancer treatments have problematic side effects. It is best to physically prepare the body for the stress that lies ahead. Aerobic and resistance training proved for me to combat these detrimental side effects. Further, patients who have been prescribed a rest-only regimen during cancer treatment typically show a 25 percent decrease in functional capacity during an eight-week treatment program.

By providing cancer patients with a higher functional capacity, a pretreatment exercise program can allay the effects of fatigue and thereby lead to an improved mood, quality of life, and treatment compliance.

Additional benefits of pretreatment fitness training extend beyond the maintenance of physical capacity. They also provide assurance that a preconditioned patient will be able to engage in physical activity both during and after treatment. Among these benefits are the preservation of cardiopulmonary function, mobility, muscle and bone strength, and psychological well-being, all of which are adversely affected by cancer therapy.

Selected Research and Studies on Exercise and Cancer

Research shows that regular exercise improves mood, body image, self-concept, and sleep patterns. Patients who exercise have a significantly better quality of life than patients who do not. Several studies have examined the relationship of exercise, rehabilitation, and quality of life in cancer patients, and they have reported positive findings.

Though there are many reasons for being physically active during cancer treatment, each person's exercise program should be based on what is safe, effective, and enjoyable for that person. Exercises should take into account any exercise program already being followed, what the individual can do now, and any physical problems or limits present. Exercise physiologists, trainers familiar with cancer patients, and oncologists and medical personnel familiar with the particular needs of cancer patients often are sources of insight into what to pursue.

Cancer experts say the shift in thinking began in the mid-1980s, coinciding with a greater awareness of health and fitness. Oncologists were faced with questions about exercise that they had never heard before. How much was allowable and when?

In the past eight years a dearth of research has become a flood of studies. Among them is one sponsored by the National Cancer Institute in 2006 that looked at the effects of moderate exercise on groups of breast and prostate cancer patients undergoing radiation therapy for six weeks.

Those assigned to a daily program—taking walks of increasing distance and doing exercises with a resistance band—had less fatigue, greater strength, and better aerobic capacity than those who were not instructed to exercise. These findings and similar ones have been replicated many times.

The American College of Sports Medicine, another national body, has weighed in on the role of exercise for helping in the cancer treatment process. In recent guidelines experts advise exercise during and after cancer treatment. Of course, each patient needs to proceed at his or her comfort level and with guidance from experienced and trained personnel. Overexertion could lead to setbacks and frustration.

Other studies indicate that moderate exercise has additional benefits, like strengthened immune function and lower rates of recurrence. Studies at Dana-Farber found that nonmetastatic colon cancer patients who routinely exercised had a 50 percent lower mortality rate during the study period than their inactive peers regardless of how active they were before the diagnosis.

The American Cancer Society (ACS) recommends that adults with cancer exercise for at least thirty minutes on most days of the week. Research, according to ACS, strongly suggests that exercise is not only safe during cancer treatment but can also improve physical functioning and quality of life.

Moderate exercise has been shown to raise self-esteem and to decrease fatigue and anxiety. It also helps with heart and blood vessel fitness, muscle strength, and body composition. People getting chemotherapy and radiation may need to exercise at a lower intensity for a time and build up more slowly than people who are not getting cancer treatment. The main goal should be to stay as active as possible.

Of course, there are certain issues for cancer survivors that may prevent or affect their ability to exercise. Some effects of treatment may increase the risk of exercise-related problems.

Where Can I Exercise?

In response to recent studies that found exercise to be beneficial in combating the effects of cancer, gyms and fitness centers have begun stepping in to meet a small but growing demand for programs designed not only to hasten the recovery of cancer patients but also to address the fatigue of chemotherapy, the swelling of lymphedema, and the loss of muscle tone.

A new program from the YMCA in partnership with the Lance Armstrong Foundation offers cancer fitness classes at more than a dozen YMCAs in ten states. At the women's gym Curves International researchers from Fox Chase Cancer Center in Philadelphia are looking at whether overweight breast cancer patients can keep to a five-day-a-week Curves routine for six months. And survivors are organizing their own classes.

In some cases oncologists are prescribing exercise and gently prodding patients to tackle whatever activity they can manage—light walking, simple stretches, and exercise with resistance bands. Yet every recommendation has its caveats. There will be days during treatment when meaningful activity is not possible, oncologists say, and that's fine. The American Cancer Society promotes moderate exercise but encourages patients to discuss their exercise plans with their oncologists and lists on its Web site (cancer.org/docroot/MIT/MIT_0.asp) thirteen precautions.

The local gym is not the only option as far as exercising is concerned. One can exercise at home, in the office, or on the way to work. It is important that it is enjoyable and stimulating so the patient will exercise regularly and not just as a passing fad. Although it is important to increase physical activity in routine activities of daily living, it is also useful to incorporate exercise into our hobbies and social life to ensure it is truly maintained for the long run.

In some geographic areas there are increasing opportunities in addition to the local gym for cancer patients and survivors to engage in exercise programs specifically designed for the cancer patient, including specific ones for specific cancers. These programs are often free. For example, my local YMCA offers a progressive exercise program for breast cancer survivors. One of the classes is a water-based rehabilitation class focused on reducing pain caused by treatment, medication, and the cancer. Another class is a land-based class emphasizing muscular strength and endurance for performing functional activities. Yet another program available for cancer patients in Southern California is End Results, a health and wellness center. Cancer patients can work out for free under the tutelage of a well-trained and focused staff.

Do you not know that in a race all the runners run, but only one receives the prize? So run that you may obtain it.
—1 Corinthians 9:24 ESV

The Power of Humor

Laughter in and of itself cannot cure cancer nor prevent cancer, but laughter as part of the full range of positive emotions including hope, love, faith, strong will to live, determination and purpose, can be a significant and indispensable aspect of the total fight for recovery.
—Dr. Harold H. Benjamin
Founder of The Wellness Community

I have found that being able to laugh at myself as well as with others has enabled me to face reality in a more positive and uplifting way. Thanks to friends who share humorous stories with me, I not only feel better but can move forward with a sense of equanimity. Humor allows an escape from the fears and stressors of the moment.

Having cancer isn't funny. It is a serious, life-changing, life-threatening occurrence. However, I have found that it has been well worth the effort to include humor into my daily life. Once I learned to live with the diagnosis and treatment, humor was extremely beneficial. A good laugh relieved stress for everyone, including me and those close to me.

Author Norman Cousins was the first to document the physiological benefits of laughter, giving validity to the adage that laughter is the best medicine. In 1964, Cousins was diagnosed with a painful and degenerative connective tissue disease and given a one-in-five-hundred chance of recovering. He theorized that if stress and negative emotions could increase the body's susceptibility to illness, then surely laughter and positive emotions could improve the body's ability to heal. Cousins discovered that ten minutes of good "belly laughter" seemed to have an anesthetic effect on him, allowing him two or more hours of pain-free sleep. He began watching Marx Brothers comedies and *Candid Camera* episodes for his self-prescribed daily doses of laughter. Cousins eventually laughed himself back to health, beating the odds and making a full recovery.

Cousins so firmly believed in the benefits of laughter that he obtained private funds to launch a pilot study investigating the healing power of humor. In this study led by Lee Berk, associate director at the Center for Neuroimmunology at Loma Linda University Medical Center, patients' blood was monitored before, during, and after sessions of mirthful laughter. They found that laughter could reduce stress hormone levels and increase the secretion of growth hormone, an enhancer of key immune responses. Dr. Berk explained, "The biological effects of a single one-hour session of viewing a humorous video can last from 12 to 24 hours, while ... daily 30-minute exposure to such humor and laughter videos produces profound and long-lasting changes in these measures." Laughter is not a cure-all, and Dr. Berk does not suggest that patients discontinue their medications or other treatments.

The use of humor is widespread in the oncologist-patient relationship and in patient literature. For example, in the January 20, 2005, issue of the *Journal of Clinical Oncology*, an article by Joshua, Cotroneo, and Clarke titled "Humor and Oncology" reinforces what Norman Cousins advanced almost seventy-five years earlier. They point out from their research and review of multiple studies that "humor serves many roles for the patient, their family, and the treating physician."

"When you make me laugh, I'm not depressed anymore!" Jerry Aragon states in his article "The Positive and Healing Power of Humor." "Professionals tell us that there can only be one emotion occupying one space at any given time. Therefore ... you're either happy or you're sad." Yet even when an individual is emotionally spent or dealing with an illness that has one facing uncertainty, humor oftentimes lifts the spirit and enables an individual, even for a short time, to cope with the situation.

George Bernard Shaw wrote, "Life does not cease to be funny when someone dies, as it does not cease to be serious when people laugh." I would modify this by saying, "Life does not cease to be funny when someone has cancer, as it does not cease to be serious when people laugh." Dr. Bernie Siegel, a cancer surgeon, wrote, "Show me a patient who is able to laugh and play, who enjoys living, and I'll show you someone who is going to live longer. Laughter makes the unbearable bearable, and a patient with a well-developed sense of humor has a better chance of recovery than a stolid individual who seldom laughs."

Definition of Humor

As the American poet e.e. Cummings wrote, "The most wasted of all days is one without laughter." Laughter is said to be a natural stress reliever. It increases the release of endorphins, the body's natural protection against depression and pain.

There is no universally accepted definition of humor and certainly not one that can reflect the subtleties in a dynamic doctor-patient relationship. In fact, the word *humor* can be used to refer to a stimulus (a comedy film), a mental process (a perception or creation of amusing incongruities), or a response (laughter or exhilaration).

In the context of oncologic care, the Association for Applied and Therapeutic Humor provides a useful definition, which defines therapeutic humor as

> "...any intervention that promotes health and wellness by stimulation of a playful discovery, expression, or appreciation of the absurdity or incongruity of life's situations. This intervention may enhance health or be used as a complementary treatment of illness to facilitate healing or coping, whether physical, emotional, cognitive, or spiritual."

Classification of Humor

Practically the classification of humor in oncology falls into two broad categories. First there is the general repartee, both planned and spontaneous, during a conversation occurring between an oncology professional and a patient or the patient's family. Secondly there is a large body of prepared humor, often found in patient literature that is generally designed to make patients see the lighter side of many aspects of cancer care.

What Is the Evidence to Date?

Current research is confirming what biblical wisdom told us centuries ago. Laughter *is* good for us. Proverbs 17:22 observed, "A cheerful heart is a good medicine, but a downcast spirit dries up the bones." The mind, body, soul, and emotions are not separate from one another but are in union. Around the seventeenth century ideas were propagated that separated the mind from the body. Unfortunately modern medicine developed from this separation concept. Now medicine is slowly returning to the holistic concept (oneness) instead of a dualistic concept (separateness).

Indiana State University College of Nursing in Terre Haute, Indiana and the University of South Florida in Tampa, Florida in 2006 reported that they found that "it is difficult to determine the relationship to any specific disease process. Whereas relationships between sense of humor and self-reported measures of physical well-being appear to be supported, more research is required to determine interrelationships between sense of humor and well-being."

According to the American Cancer Society, "Complementary methods are defined as supportive methods used to complement evidence-based treatment. Complementary therapies do not replace mainstream cancer treatment and are not promoted to cure disease. Rather, they control symptoms and improve well-being and quality of life." Alternative therapies or alternative medicine by contrast involve nonmainstream treatments that patients sometimes use in place of orthodox treatments. Taken together, these therapies are known as complementary and alternative medicine or CAM. Humor falls within the CAM definition when used as a component of an alternative treatment.

Per an article appearing in a 1987 issue of *Psychology Today*, "If stress and negative emotions can suppress the immune system, why can't laughter and feelings of trust and hope promote healing, even prolong life?" Laughter is believed to act as a coping mechanism to reduce stress, improve self-esteem, and reduce psychological symptoms related to negative life events.

A sense of humor, measured by several different self-reporting instruments, is correlated with increased self-esteem and decreased depressive personality attributes. Although relationships between sense of humor and depression or depressive personality appear to be supported by the available literature, more research is needed to determine whether this demonstrates the effect of sense of humor on depression or the effect of depression on sense of humor. Controlled, focused research is indisputably needed.

The Powers of Humor and Laughter

It is sad that the ones who enjoy humor, laughter, fun, and play to the fullest are young children. Most adults become far too serious. Children tend to laugh an average of four hundred times a day. For adults, a recent laughter study shows that 64 percent of people smile less than twenty times a day at home, and 72 percent smile less than twenty times a day at work. The International Congress of Humor found that laughter is down 66 to 82 percent worldwide compared to what it was in the 1950s. In the 1950s people laughed an average of eighteen minutes a day. Today the average is between four to six minutes a day.

Earlier I mentioned that when I was in my hospital room a few hours after a surgery, I had a moment of panic when I woke up somewhat in a fog. Without my glasses, I was definitely not able to see with much clarity—not that it would have made much difference at the time. I heard the alarm of what proved to be the machine that provides the drip, drip, drip nourishment through one of the feeding tubes. The noise was incessant and magnified in my mind. No one was coming to help me, and I was certain that the noise was emanating from a heart monitor connected to me!

As I felt around the bed for the apparatus that contained the button to press to call the nursing station, my heart raced. Finally I had something on my chest, and there was a button on it, which I pressed. Several times I pressed it, and that was all that

I remembered. Later—how much later I didn't know—I woke up to experience the same emotions and repeated my search to press the button.

Three times I had the same experience.

Finally I woke up, and a very nice nurse was standing beside the bed. She was changing the bag of liquid refreshment that was being pumped into my body. She also reset the machine—the pump—and the noise stopped.

When I asked about the instrument on my chest that I had pressed the button on to call the nursing station, my nurse informed me that it actually was for use if I felt any pain and would provide me with a shot of morphine! The maximum at any given time was three releases of the morphine.

To this day, my wife and I still laugh about my experience and how I put myself back to sleep so easily!

Jokes on the Internet may initiate a chuckle, but it is not the same as the belly-jiggling, rib-tickling laughter reaction when there is interaction with others. Socializing with friends and relatives has been drastically reduced in recent times for many people. Humor and laughter in the workplace have eroded as well.

I know that laughing makes me feel better emotionally, but now scientific studies are also revealing positive physiological effects. Humor and laughter can

- *reduce pain* by triggering the pituitary gland to secrete endorphins, a natural painkiller;
- *stimulate the immune system* to fight infection;
- *give a feeling of well-being* brought on when the endocrine system secretes hormones called catecholamines;
- *aid brain function* by improving circulation and oxygenating the body; and
- *improve discernment* by stimulating the hypothalamus.

Humor is an antidote to all ills. I believe that fun is as important as love. Humor has made my life joyous and fun. It can do the same for you. Find something to laugh at every day. Cancer is not a death sentence any longer. It is a wake-up call about mutations of cells that are out of control.

Mirth is God's medicine. Everybody ought to bathe in it.
—Henry Ward Beecher
Clergyman, social reformer, abolitionist, and speaker

The Power of Touch

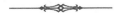

Too often we underestimate the power of touch, a smile, a kind word, a listening ear, an honest compliment, or the smallest act of caring, all of which have the potential to turn a life around.

—Leo F. Buscaglia
Author, motivational speaker, and professor

Touch is to most people almost as necessary to life as air, water, and food. Yet for others the very thought of being touched by strangers often sends chills up their spines. The latter was true for me. Touches or hugs were fine for my wife, but having others touch my body was off limits.

Once many years ago Marty gave me a gift certificate to have a massage. She was overjoyed that I consented to try it, and the big day arrived.

I lasted less than five minutes.

The masseuse, who was extremely professional, slowly walked me through the process, and then I lay down on the massage table. The masseuse began to touch my back and asked if the pressure was too much. I said no, but my body was screaming inside that this didn't feel right. Some of my emotional baggage— unpleasant memories long repressed from my youth—kicked in. I wasn't prepared for my reaction, which was immediate—that this experience, which was intended to be soothing and helpful, represented pain and suffering.

The anguish that was building up inside was overwhelming. It continued as the masseuse massaged my back. Finally I sat up, said, "Thank you," to the masseuse, and said that we were done.

She was alarmed that something had been done either to hurt me or to cause me to question her abilities, so I took a few minutes to explain that the massage was not my thing and that I no longer wanted to continue. With that, I put my clothes back on, bounded out of the room, the masseuse following me to the front desk, gave her a tip, and went home.

With the passage of time and as a consequence of my own personal journey, the idea of being touched has taken on a whole different meaning.

With my wife's stroke more than a decade and a half ago, priorities changed because of the fact that literally and figuratively "in a blink of an eye" our lives changed dramatically. Her stroke led us to a place in our minds where we examined and determined what was vital to us. No longer did our careers seem so important. Neither did the mundane sameness of daily living.

Marty's stay in the hospital's ICU unit was a very traumatic time for me, seeing my wife holding onto life, with tubes monitoring her every breath and providing nourishment, watching the monitors bleeping, and experiencing the code-blue medical team rushing into her room on at least three occasions and clearing out visitors. It was very apparent that things had changed.

Into our lives came friends—some old and some new—who held onto me or, when they could, tightly squeezed my wife's hand or touched her arm or leg. Some patted her lovely head of hair—now in disarray, yet to me it was as beautiful as it had always been. Once she was moved to the acute rehabilitation hospital with her "weaknesses"—cognitive and physical—she and I held onto each other tightly and shared tender moments of touching and talking. We did this despite the fact that her speech was slurred, her face distorted as if she had Bell's palsy. One eye was almost completely shut, and one arm, one leg, and one hand were very weak.

We connected on a very touching level that we had not experienced for many years, and it brought a new understanding to me of the power of touch. Just as we as children look for hugs when we fall and scrape our knees, we as adults crave to be touched or to touch those in need. In our situation the experience of hugging for long periods of time was emotional, exhilarating, and most meaningful.

As I mentioned previously, our son flew down immediately from the Seattle area when he heard of his mother's stroke. Our daughter, who was due to deliver her firstborn, came to be at her mother's side to add physical and emotional support, surrounding us with love and hope. This was a turning point in all of our lives.

Marty went on to spend several weeks in an acute rehabilitation hospital specializing in strokes, where she was determined to do whatever it took to become mobile and as good as she could be. After she returned to our home, she immediately spent five days a week and eight hours a day in various therapy experiences for another eleven and a half months, and since then she has continued to have a "new normal" experience.

I found that human touch is as life-sustaining as air, water, and food. Babies need to be held by parents. As adults, we need to be touched as well, whether it comes from a friendly hug or an embrace or reaching out and caressing a loved one's hair.

The power of touch is enormous. I keep repeating this because I discovered how important it is.

Just imagine never being touched—no hand on the shoulder, no pat on the back, no physical link with any other living thing!

The simple act of touching, not necessarily in a sexual manner, is so powerful that it can, according to many health studies, slow the heart rate, decrease blood pressure, and strengthen the immune system. American culture is not very affectionate, and I believe that we are losing out on the benefits of regular physical interaction with others.

What is it about touch that makes it so valuable to life? The skin is the largest organ of our body, a shield from external harm, and a key to sexual interaction. It is a pathway through which touch is translated into something meaningful.

While our other four senses (sight, hearing, smell, and taste) are located in specific parts of the body, our sense of touch is found all over the body. This is because the sense of touch originates in the bottom layer of the skin called the dermis. The dermis is filled with tiny nerve endings that give information about the things with which body comes in contact. The information is transmitted to the spinal cord, which sends messages to the brain, where the feeling is registered. Experiencing the world through our senses is the way we as humans often process information that is useful to us. Imagine a world without sight, hearing, smell, taste, or touch. Even if we lost only one of our five senses, it would be a much less enjoyable world.

The nerve endings in skin can tell if something is hot or cold, smooth or rough. They can also feel if something causes pain. The body has about twenty different types of nerve endings that send messages to our brain. However, the most common receptors are heat, cold, pain, pressure, and touch receptors. Pain receptors are probably the most important for our safety because they protect us by warning our brain that the body is hurt!

Some areas of the body are more sensitive than others because they have more nerve endings. Have you ever bitten your tongue and wondered why it hurt so much? It is because the sides of our tongue have a lot of nerve endings that are very sensitive to pain.

However, the tongue is not as good at sensing hot or cold. That is why it is easy to burn the mouth when we eat something really hot. Fingertips are also very sensitive. For example, most people who are blind use their fingertips to read Braille by feeling the patterns of raised dots on paper. Safecrackers have been known to sand fingertips for even greater sensitivity.

It is my opinion that people thrive when touched, but some people do not get touched enough. It is true that there are quite a number of people who do not know how uptight they are until someone touches them. It can be like a massive sigh released from the body by that touch. Sadly touch may often dwindle as individuals' age. Children may feel awkward hugging a frail frame or shy away from kissing Grandma's cheeks. Older people are just younger ones in older bodies. People may feel like the same person at twelve or seventy, even if a little stiffer or slower. Older men have been known to touch their spouses less as they age because of diminished or nonexistent sexual ability. It is in this later time of life that the need for physical contact with a loved one may be the greatest. Imagine how you would feel if no one ever touched you with care again!

Children instinctively initiate and seek out touch when they need or want it. As people age, sometimes there is less giving and receiving of touch for a variety of reasons. At times touch is equated with sexuality. Some individuals carry baggage of abuse from the past. It is easy to forget that touch is needed as much as or more than when we were youngsters. Some rationalize that touch isn't important. Part of this may be to cover up hurt from our past if we grew up in families that didn't touch one another.

Yet though younger individuals may ignore the older generation who may be silently crying out for contact, animals make no such discrimination. Dogs, for example, may stimulate elderly individuals. Some research shows that interaction with several kinds of animals reduces stress.

I firmly believe that the sense of touch and feeling are at the very core of our being, of the body-mind-soul connection.

Science tells us that a touch triggers the release of brain endorphins, an endogenous analgesic that may be more powerful than heroin or morphine. But touch is more than just a scientific confluence of brain chemicals according to Michael G. Rayel in "First Aid to Mental Illness," (Soar Dime, 2008). Perhaps there is more to hugging and touching than just the release of endorphins. Touch provides comfort. It makes us feel secure because it unites us with an affectionate, loving, and feeling human being. The warmth it brings may be better than the warmth a fireplace can provide. A touch may make the body resistant to stress. Indeed, touch is the best remedy, and it's free.

When my wife hugs me at night, I can feel all my aches and concerns of the day disappear instantly. I feel refreshed and transformed. I feel recharged, a dynamo ready to capture dreams and to take risks. When I come home after a full day's work and my kids hug me, I feel an immediate relief. I then celebrate joyfully.

Research on Touch

There are bumper stickers asking, "Have you hugged your child today?" Apparently the bumper sticker reflects the fact that the driver and others are recognizing the need for touch. Furthermore, YouTube video clips on the need for hugs from various locations around the globe provide another reminder of the need for touch.

The Cleveland Clinic, based on its own 2010 research and experience with patients, indicates that the mind-body connection means that people can learn to use thoughts positively to influence some of the body's physical responses, thereby decreasing or increasing stress responses. Remembering a happy experience triggers the body and mind to relax. Recalling an upsetting or frightening experience may make the heart beat faster. Sweating may accompany this experience, and hands may become cold and clammy as well.

Whether a patient has been diagnosed with an illness such as cancer or has a need to prepare for a medical procedure like surgery, it is very important to minimize negative effects and maximize the healthy, healing aspects of the mind–body connection.

At the Cleveland Clinic and other medical facilities, a variety of calming and empowering mind–body exercises have been proven to help people accomplish the following:

- decrease anxiety
- decrease pain
- enhance sleep
- decrease the use of medication for post-surgical pain
- decrease side effects of medical procedures
- reduce recovery time and shorten hospital stays
- strengthen the immune system and enhance the ability to heal
- increase sense of control and well-being

Other medical institutions, such as Cincinnati Children's Hospital, Stanford University, the Institute for Postgraduate Dental Education in Sweden, and the University of Iowa, use research findings on touch to improve physical and psychological states. Methods such as Reiki and Tui na are hands-on body treatments that are also being studied for their beneficial effects.

Reiki is a Japanese technique for stress reduction and relaxation that also promotes healing. It is performed by "laying on hands" and is based on the idea that an unseen life-force energy flows through us and is what causes us to be alive. If our life-force energy is low, then we are more likely to get sick or feel stress, and if it is high, we are more capable of being happy and healthy. The word *Reiki* is made of two Japanese words—*Rei*, which means "God's wisdom" or "the Higher Power," and *ki*, which is "life-force energy." So Reiki is actually "spiritually guided life force energy." Tui na (or acupressure) involves pressure by the hands on the same points on the body used during acupuncture.

A pilot study involving men with localized prostate cancer and women with advanced cervical cancer has begun to see whether touch can boost the immune system and improve the body's natural defenses against the disease. Work at Duke University in Durham, North Carolina, has shown that touch and massage can cut levels of stress hormones and may also increase levels of melatonin and the feel-good hormone, serotonin.

Researchers at Ohio State University have found that wounds took a day longer to heal when the patient had been involved in an argument with a loved one, and that in married couples who did not get along well wound healing took two days longer. "Wounds in the couples who were hostile healed at only 60 per cent of the rate of couples with low levels of hostility," said Dr. Janice Kiecolt-Glaser.

At DePauw University in Indiana Dr. Matthew Hertenstein discovered that touch communicates emotions. When people were touched by a stranger they could not see but who had been instructed to try to communicate a particular emotion, they were able to tell the emotional state of the other person with great accuracy.

Dr. Hertenstein said, "Our study is the first to provide rigorous evidence showing that humans can reliably signal love, gratitude and sympathy with touch. These findings raise the interesting possibility that touch may convey more positive emotions than the face."

"It [touch] is the first language we learn," states Dacher Keltner, a professor of psychology at the University of California, Berkeley, and the author of *Born to Be Good: The Science of a Meaningful Life*. Touch remains, he said, "our richest means of emotional expression throughout life."

Another study on the subject titled "Brief Report: Autistic Children's Attentiveness and Responsivity Improve after Touch Therapy" in the *Journal of Autism and Developmental Disorders* found that a sympathetic touch from a doctor leaves people with the impression that the visit lasted twice as long compared with estimates from people who were untouched. Research by Tiffany Field of the Touch Research Institute in Miami has found that a massage from a loved one can not only ease pain but also soothe depression and strengthen a relationship.

The metaphors of "being touched by his words" and "touched by the act of kindness" imply that both the mind and the body *feel*. Others touch one's life. People say, "Let's keep in touch." All of these things indicate how important touch is. The laying on of hands originates in the Bible (Acts 13:3).

How Touch Helped Me in Treatment

I learned up close and personal that undergoing an MRI increased my anxiety as well as my claustrophobia. Magnetic resonance imaging (MRI) is a diagnostic technique that uses a magnetic field to produce pictures of structures inside the body. During an MRI, your body is in a very strong magnetic field. The MRI machine also uses pulses of radio waves. The machine creates an image based on the way hydrogen atoms in your body react to the magnetic field and the radio waves. Usually images are created of several slices, like those in a loaf of bread, of an organ or part of the body. The MRI's computer also can combine these slices into three-dimensional (3-D) images.

Because water molecules are especially sensitive to the forces used in this technique, MRI scans are very good at showing differences in water content between different body tissues. This is particularly important in detecting tumors and in checking for problems in the body's soft tissues, such as the brain, spinal cord, heart, and eye.

MRI is a painless technique (unless you are claustrophobic) that usually takes about twenty minutes. The patient lies on a scanning table. If a cylindrical scanner is being used, the table will slide through the narrow opening into the MRI cylinder. In an open MRI the table will slide so that the part of the body being scanned is surrounded by the scanning element, or the machine will move over the patient on the table. The patient will periodically hear very loud knocking noises as the scanner works. The technicians operating the machine will be in another room, but they talk to the patient through speakers in the machine or through earphones.

The first time that I had to enter a closed MRI machine was a traumatic experience, as I am extremely claustrophobic. Even with the aid of an antianxiety pill, I found myself walking into the room where the machine was located with my heart rate as well as my fear increased a hundredfold.

The members of the technical staff were as understanding and professional as one could ever desire. They put me on the scanning table and slowly explained what was going to happen in very soothing and quiet voices. I received an explanation for what was being done each step of the way. As soon as the mask was placed over my head, I announced, "I will be still. Don't tie me down." It was a control thing!

The staff reluctantly went along with my wishes, and I was slowly moved on what became in my mind a conveyor belt into this very dark, long tunnel with no light at the end of it! If there was no light, it meant to my mind that there was a train coming at me from the other end of the tunnel, and we were on a collision course.

"You're doing great," came the voice out of the machine. "How are you feeling?"

"Hurry up!" I said excitedly and fearfully. A small motion occurred, signaling slight progress. Within seconds I yelled out, "Get me out of here!"

The voice responded quickly. "You're doing great. We only have about an hour more to go, and we have just begun."

"If you don't get me out of this machine *now*, I am going to break it!" I yelled at the top of my lungs. The machine's whirring noise came to a slow halt as I was slowly placed in reverse on the conveyer belt, and I quickly bolted off of it. The time that had elapsed was about ninety seconds.

After some discussion it was decided that a few more little pink pills and about fifteen to twenty minutes of quiet time would enable me to endure the procedure easily. I was given a time-out and sent to a room where Marty and I sat quietly. Soon—too soon for my fearful state of mind—we were invited to go back to the MRI room. I looked at the machine, my eyes wide open, my heart racing, and I stated emphatically that there was no way that I was getting back into that machine. The antianxiety drugs had had the opposite of their intended effect on me, and I was in no mood to undergo that traumatic event again.

A week later with my wife by my side, I had an open MRI. It took a few of those little pink pills (lorazepam) to reduce my anxiety, and the medical team allowed Marty to be in the room with me. It was an unorthodox MRI, and the machine was not one that could get the best of pictures; however, I was able to get through it. Why? My wife's presence in the room and her being able to hold my hand throughout the ordeal comforted me and helped get me through it. (I may have publically been a self-assured and always-in-control person, and yet behind closed doors—the doors of an MRI room—I was a wimp who needed my wife to hold my hand!)

When the MRI was finished after an exceedingly long time, the technician came to me, holding some towels. He handed me one and said, "You may want to use this and dry off." I wondered why and then looked down. I saw that my pants looked like I had an accident that had covered them. It was perspiration. The technician was using the rest of the towels to dry off the bed of the MRI machine, as it was soaking wet from my perspiration as well!

As my cancer journey continues, there are more scans and MRIs, all being part of the protocols for qualifying for and fulfilling the requirements of the experimental clinical trials. I am able, thanks in large measure to Marty and her serenity and touch, to have considerably less fear and anxiety and more peace as I submit the various imaging tools needed to assess my condition.

The Healing Power of Touch

In the health field, the healing touch evokes an emotional response. Read this story and recognize that although it is several years old, it still rings true today:

> In recent years, a 40-year-old man was hospitalized for treatment of advanced leukemia. While he was receiving massive doses of chemotherapy, he was put in quarantine for fear that even catching a common cold from family or friends could be potentially lethal. During isolation, his family could come no closer than his door, and then had to stand separated from him with masks covering their mouths. The only person allowed to touch the patient

was a nurse who had been specially cleared as being in good health.

Here is how the patient described the experience of isolation: "This nurse changed my bedding and kept me clean and all that," he said. "But she hated to touch me, or at least it felt that way. Whatever she was doing she did with as little physical contact as possible."

"I wish I could have told her how important touch was," he added. "I craved the feeling of flesh on flesh. I craved it! It wasn't a sexual thing—in my condition that was the last thing on my mind. But I really felt I was losing my will to live without that touch. I mean, I still wanted to live, to get better, but the reason to keep struggling was slipping away from me. I needed the feeling of someone's skin on mine to help me find it again."

This story appeared in the November–December 1991 issue of *American Fitness*. It was told by Victor M. Parachin in "The Healing Power of Touch: The Simple Act of Touching Frequently Reduces Everyday Anxiety and Tension."

"People who are more comfortable with touch are less afraid and less suspicious of other people's motives and intentions," says Stephen Thayer, professor of psychology at the City University of New York.

According to Gretchen Malik in "The Healing Power of Touch" (Suite 101.com, 2001), women appreciate touches because their skin is more sensitive than men's. Malik also said that babies who are not touched fail to grow normally. Children, she states, who are not lovingly touched often grow up to be more physically violent. And that's a shame because our society is starting to become a "hands to ourselves" environment.

In her book *Healing with Heart*, Terri Moss writes about a patient who had recently undergone surgery for cancer. The patient found the operating room to be cold and sterile. This added to his already anxious state. Then one of the nurses touched his arm, and another stroked his hair. This human touch reassured him and put him at ease. He later told a nurse, "I want you to know how important that was."

Mother Teresa discovered the power of touch when she said that more than hunger, poverty, and physical suffering, it is the lack of love that makes people die every day. She used to touch the lepers and bathe their wounds with her own hands.

Power of Pets

Having had pets in our home, including cats, birds, snakes, hamsters, and others, the importance of pets has been an integral part of our lives, particularly when our children were in our home.

The idea of pets for therapy is becoming more common from organizations such as Delta Society, Pet Partners, Pawprints and Purrs, Love on a Leash, and PAWS, just to name a few. Whether it be dogs, cats, horses, or other animals, pets can be beneficial to health. One recent study by researchers at the State University of New York, Buffalo, looked at the effects of pet ownership on forty-eight stockbrokers who were already taking medication for hypertension. This study found that the twenty-four stockbrokers who were given a pet had a significantly better reduction in high blood pressure accompanying stress than those without pets did.

"Most studies show a direct benefit from stroking a pet, for example, but this one goes a step further in that the act of owning a pet lowered blood pressure," says Alan Entin, past president of the division of family psychology of the American Psychological Association.

"There is something about the outside of a horse that is good for the inside of a man." This famous quote, attributed to Sir Winston Churchill, definitely sets the stage as an introduction to a very significant and moving story about the healing relationships that are formed between humans and animals. Whether they are small, pampered house pets or powerful horses, it makes no difference.

Animal-assisted therapy is now used for patients not responsive to traditional treatment. For example, Dr. Ken Marten at Sea Life Park in Hawaii reports that autistic children have been known to open up and to begin communicating with dolphins.

Therapeutic horseback riding is now a recognized and mainstream treatment modality that holds great promise for widely diverse medical conditions ranging from physical disabilities to emotional, behavioral, and learning disabilities to substance abuse issues.

Nature's Corner, an Internet site "for those who are passionate about their animals and nature" indicates on its Web page, "The Healing Power of Pets," that several medical reports have credited animals with positive effects on people's lives, such as:

- lowering blood pressure and stress for everyday people
- helping people cope with the loss of a loved one and other major life changes
- improving communication in marriages
- helping people with disabilities live normal lives (through such service animals as Seeing Eye dogs)
- helping people cope with cancer, Alzheimer's, and AIDS
- correlating with higher survival rates for people with coronary heart disease
- improving young children's socialization with peers and development of nurturing behavior
- giving a sense of constancy to foster children

- improving results for anxious and depressed people
- helping to improve balance, posture, mobility, language, and muscle coordination (through therapeutic horseback riding)
- facilitating social interactions between strangers and improving social behavior for prisoners and mentally impaired people
- enabling more recreational activity, such as dog walking

When our two children were very young, Marty and I had a wonderful cat named Millie. She was a joy not only for our children but also for my wife and me. When Millie became with child, our daughter and son watched her behavior and often spent long hours caring for the cat. The night that Millie gave birth to her kittens—all six of them—both Michelle and David Jr. were there to watch the blessed event. They oohed and aahed as each kitten arrived on the scene. From that moment they seemed to enjoy Millie more and to realize how important Millie was to the total family. They also came to appreciate more fully and respect how precious the animals—the little kittens in this case—were as they grew and blossomed and finally were adopted by various families.

Little did we know that from this early experience with animals that our daughter would develop an enjoyment of animals and birds that she would carry into adulthood.

Michelle—a lovely, caring, and beautiful woman—had an African gray parrot for almost thirty-five years. The bird was originally named Messerschmitt until Michelle discovered almost twenty years later that she was a female, and then she became Mez. Mez was a constant companion of our daughter's through high school, college, marriage, and as a single woman with a son.

Michelle was so enamored with birds—at one time she had more than 125 birds in aviaries that were on our back porch, patio,

111

and backyard—that when she went off to college she immediately called herself Robin, and to this day most of her college friends know her by that name.

In sickness and health, Mez and Robin were inseparable. In fact, much trauma and drama occurred if something happened to either one, as each had a sense of the other's state of mind or state of health. Touch was a cure for both, as Mez enjoyed having her neck slowly and softly massaged. So did our daughter. Just having each other near—the touch of Mez on our daughter's shoulder, cradled in her hand, or sitting on her arm—reduced the stress and strain of everyday life. When our daughter was in pain, sick, or stressed out, Mez would whistle or try to express herself through music to indicate wanting to be held closely.

The therapeutic effect of that closeness allowed our daughter to feel, in the moment, that someone cared for her, that someone was there for her. The inner peace that came with the touch and sound of Mez enabled her to improve her outlook on getting better from her own stresses in life.

Mez recently had to be put down. The care and gentleness of the veterinarian, once the decision was made that no additional interventions would help Mez, was a difficult one. My daughter and my wife wept and consoled each other. I spent some time with Mez, stroking the back of her neck on the fateful morning when the decision was made. It was difficult for our daughter's son to see his mother in pain and to see Mez in her listless state.

Michelle held Mez until the bird died. She stroked Mez on the bird's head and neck and held on until the last breath of air departed Mez's body. It was sad. It was beautiful. It was caring. It was loving. The question is this: Who was the caregiver, and who was being cared for all of these years?

What we miss is the physical presence and interaction with our pet. However, it is comforting to know that although her physical form is gone; her passing was made as easy as possible. As guardians, it is our responsibility to assure pets a peaceful, painless death and dying process. It is a final act of love toward one that has been meaningful and integral part of a family's life.

Our daughter has lost the physical presence of her bird. However, the passing of a loved pet did not sever the bond of love. There is a legacy of cherished memories and love that transcends time and space.

The Importance of Hugs

> You can't wrap love in a box, but you
> can wrap a person in a hug.
> —Author unknown

A hug is one of the most basic ways two human beings touch. There is power in a hug.

How Hugs Can Heal

In an article in *The Independent* titled "How the Power of Touch Reduces Pain and Even Fights Disease," Roger Dobson draws attention to the role that hugging can play in the healing process. (http://www.independent.co.uk/life-style/health-and-families/health-news/how-the-power-of-touch-reduces-pain-and-even-fights-disease-419462.html). In addition, advanced understanding obtained in some cases from research includes the following insights:

* Hugging your partner could lower his or her blood pressure.

- Researchers have found that in younger women the more hugs they get, the lower their blood pressure.
- Researchers at the University of North Carolina who investigated sixty-nine premenopausal women showed that those who had the most hugs had a reduced heart rate.
- Exactly what could be responsible is not clear, but the UNC psychiatrists also found that blood levels of the hormone oxytocin were much higher in the women who were hugged the most.
- Other research finds that oxytocin is released during social contact and that it is associated with social bonding. A study at Ohio State University shows that when it is put into wounds in animals, the injuries heal much more quickly.
- Work at the Swedish University of Agricultural Sciences suggests that oxytocin can induce antistress effects, including reduction in blood pressure and levels of the stress hormone cortisol. "It increases pain thresholds and stimulates various types of positive social interaction, and it promotes growth and healing. Oxytocin can be released by various types of non-noxious sensory stimulation, for example by touch and warmth," they say.

A dear friend sent this to me from her daily calendar. She reached out and touched me with this insight: "Everyone was meant to share God's all-abiding love and care. He saw that we would need to know a way to let these feelings show. So God made hugs."

It's simple but good.

It is the magic of a touch, the power of a hug that makes life joyful.

The Power of Friendship

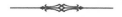

I get by with a little help from my friends.
　　　　　　　　　　　　　　　　　　—The Beatles

In previous chapters, I described how supportive my family was when I was diagnosed with cancer. Obviously each situation is different, but it is worth mentioning some of the experiences that are common for cancer patients with regard to their family and friends.

Each cancer patient has his or her own needs. The diagnosis may lead to depression, loss of appetite, irritability, anger, loss of sleep, and an inability to cope. The cancer experience can cause some patients to feel isolated or to withdraw from people who were close prior to the cancer diagnosis. Sometimes friends disappear or are unable to provide the kind of help a patient needs or wants. Cancer patients who are able to maintain social interactions with family and friends during the course of their treatment are less likely to suffer from severe depression—an extremely common problem among patients newly diagnosed with cancer.

Frequently individuals considered friends seem to become strangely absent. The reality behind this rejection may stem from an irrational fear of cancer or an unwillingness to face mortality. People simply don't know how to deal with cancer.

In some instances, individuals who had been my friends decided not to continue being around me. My initial observation was that they would shy away or keep conversation to a minimum. Telephone calls became infrequent, and invitations for lunch became a thing of the past. Soon there was no interaction at all with some people.

Initially I thought it was just my imagination. I did have more time to think about myself and friends during the long periods of time in doctors' offices and in treatment centers. It is easy to get paranoid! When I broached the subject with others who were dealing with cancer or other illnesses, they, too, had experienced similar things. Of course, some people have remained close through the trying times of treatments, side effects, and unsociability because of fatigue. I have been blessed by my circle of friends, who lift my spirits and remain a significant cheering section for my ongoing fight of beating cancer.

My friend Andrew provides another good example. Andrew's children handled his illness in two very different ways. His son, Bob, immediately became involved in the decision-making process; helping to determine what steps might be taken to help his father combat the cancer. Bob's sister was unable to come to terms with her father's illness and was almost entirely absent from Andrew's care and treatment discussions. In addition, one of Andrew's closest friends stopped talking to him not long after he was diagnosed. Another friend of Andrew's, in the course of conversation about his illness, told him to "stop being so self-absorbed." Needless to say, Andrew was confused by the treatment he received from his family and friends.

It is impossible to say what baggage others carry with them or what might cause them to react the way they do. They may be overwhelmed by what is going on in their own lives. The only things you have control of are your own actions and responses.

It does not help anyone to become judgmental regarding the reactions of others. You cannot know their motivations.

Some people do not know what to say when a friend announces he or she has been diagnosed with cancer. Friends may appear unsupportive when actually they might just be very uncomfortable with the thought of something bad happening to a relative or friend. Some people cannot manage the threat of death. My suggestion is to be open about what is going on in your life but give details only when and if the other person wants to hear all that you might tell him or her. Ask if the person has any questions. The important thing is not to give up on friends and to learn how best to accommodate awkward feelings and still maintain the friendship. Focusing on how your friend is doing adds some normalcy to the relationship.

What Is a Friend?

A friend is one who knows you as you are, understands
where you have been, accepts who you have become,
invites you to grow and supports you in your journey.
—Anonymous

The definition of a friend is different for each individual and varies as a person ages. Some friendships begin as early as grammar school and remain intact throughout life. These friendships shape personalities and values as maturity occurs. Friends influence the ability to achieve happiness and self-esteem, and they are a source of strength and energy as well. In good times and bad, people who are our genuine friends share in whatever the situation may be and will offer honest opinions and ideas for solutions to problems we encounter.

Relationships that are negative or destructive usually do not last, as they are based on goals that are detrimental. These are not real friendships.

When events occur that are significant like the diagnosis of cancer, most patients choose to take advantage of the relationships that have been meaningful. Frequently the people cancer patients reach out to are not relatives but individuals who have become friends in the past. Distance and time are not relevant where friends are concerned.

Some associations develop over a long period of time, and others are almost instant. Best friends forever (BFFs) are the unique contacts who may be the most significant, especially in periods of difficulties. There is no question that genuine friendships are gifts beyond compare. They can bring and have brought me deep peace and satisfaction.

Being Kind to Self and Others

> That best portion of a good man's life? His little,
> nameless, unremembered acts of kindness and of love.
> —William Wordsworth
> English poet

Ultimately kindness is deep caring.

Kindness is exhibited through thoughts and actions. It basically involves respect.

Understand that someone you feel may have abandoned you might have commitments beyond your knowledge that limit the time for contact with you. There may be people to whom you as the cancer patient must extend additional effort to preserve what you assumed previously was a true friendship. Sometimes the kind thing to do is to reach out again and again to others, even when your perception is that they have deserted you. Others may be waiting for contact from you, as they may not want to drain the energy you have left following treatments and therapies. They could be dealing with something totally unknown to you and might welcome a call from you.

Being kind is also asking friends what is going on in their lives and not focusing totally on the difficulties you are experiencing with cancer. This also shows that you as a friend are interested in them and not just looking for support from them. Again, keep in mind that those you come in contact with also have limits to their time and energy and that these may be factors in time spent with you.

The Importance of Friends

> As the sun makes ice melt, kindness causes
> misunderstanding, mistrust, and hostility to evaporate.
> —Albert Schweitzer
> French philosopher, theologian,
> organist, physician, and medical missionary

Friends make our lives better. Distance does not separate friends, and as I have mentioned in previous chapters, some of my best friends live in various parts of the country and world. I have learned never to take friendships for granted.

As children, some of us had imaginary friends or beloved pets who became our intimate pals that were available to listen to our dreams and secrets. Friends are a big part of forming our personalities and shaping who we become through our teens and into our adult lives. As we age, illness and injury add some unexpected layers to our lives. Friends support one another during difficult times.

A recent study by Pennsylvania State University revealed that men and women react differently to stress in the way they behave socially. Men have a tendency either to go off by themselves or to engage in a highly competitive sport with other men. Women seek one another out and commiserate. A nurses' health study at the Harvard Medical School concluded that for women not having friends was as bad for their health as obesity or smoking. In fact, friendships can help us live longer, and they can most definitely help us manage stress. Because friends accept us for who we are, we gain the confidence to dream great dreams. We can even trust them with our most embarrassing secrets!

For cancer patients, one of the most important factors in recovery is the understanding and acceptance of friends. Friends can make a difference by offering reassurance, companionship, and emotional strength.

As mentioned earlier, we have different kinds of friends in different parts of our lives, but not all friendships last forever. However, they are parts of our lives and our memories. While we are building a friendship, we learn and benefit from our friends through their encouragement, affection, support, trust, and kindness. When we have a good relationship with someone, it makes us feel happy and joyful. Friendship makes us more human, as it helps us to realize that others have the same needs as we do and how friendship fulfills them. In the end, friendship helps us to see how precious life is and why we are living.

Why We Need Friends

> Don't walk in front of me; I may not follow.
> Don't walk behind me; I may not lead.
> Just walk beside me and be my friend.
>
> —Albert Campus
> French author, journalist, and philosopher

As modern technology increases our access to other people, our intimate relationships may become scarcer. Families are smaller, and relatives don't necessarily live in close proximity anymore. More individuals work from home with the use of computers, eliminating the opportunity for personal contacts in an office setting.

That same modern technology that permits easy connections with people from all over the world also tends to get in the way of time spent in face-to-face relationships. Text and e-mail have replaced telephone calls and human interactions.

"You have cancer" may be the most loaded sentence in the English language. As soon as an individual hears those words, the mind may conjure frightening thoughts of pain, suffering, and death. In order to deal effectively and courageously with this major illness, cancer patients need not only medical care but also the resolute support of friends. Friends are helpful in delivering encouragement and inspiration to one another.

"A friend is one who believes in you when you have ceased to believe in yourself." This anonymous quote aptly describes the role that a friend plays in your life. Friends are the ones who are always there for you, whether the times are good or bad. Words are not necessary when in the presence of a friend.

In short, friends are important because, among other things, they are always there for you, laugh with you in the happy times, give you a shoulder when you cry, serve as one of the biggest supports in your life, accept you as you are, will never lie to you, can be counted on always, make you feel special, will offer advice and be truthful when you ask for it, care for you.

Additionally, friends are the ones with whom darkest secrets can be shared without fear of secrets being divulged, feel happy at your success, commiserate with your difficulties, and eliminate any feelings of loneliness you might possess.

Don't underestimate the value of new contacts that cancer patients will make through support groups. Will Rogers said, "A stranger is just a friend I haven't met yet."

People are like stars ... we all have our own special light
that shines from within. Sometimes we find our light to
be dim and we struggle to shine ... but that is when we
need the light shed from the other stars to help us light
our path once again. A true light that comes from within,
from our divine Maker is so brilliant that it penetrates into
the souls of the other stars onto which it shines, leaving its
impression for eternity. Are you shining for someone today?
—Anonymous

The Power of Hope

With communication comes understanding and clarity.
With understanding, fear diminishes.
In the absence of fear, hope emerges.
And in the presence of hope, anything is possible.

—Ellen Stovall
Cancer survivor of more than thirty years

One of the paradoxes of the human condition is that even though we know we are mortals, we wish those we love could live forever. We also wish our own lives could be lived out with less pain, suffering, uncertainty, and fear. But incurable diseases know no boundaries of geography, religion, race, or ethnicity. Life-altering sicknesses eventually make their presence felt in our lives, forcing unexpected changes.

The ways we react to these changes vary with each culture and with each family. In the past decade new advances in medical technology have made it possible to live longer with serious diseases, and they have also complicated the choices we have in treatment. Collectively these new realities have impacted the ways communities, families, and individuals are responding to illness.

When you are facing cancer, you want answers. You want hope. And you want both at the same time.

For many people it is hard to imagine being presented with the life-changing words "You have cancer." Yet every day thousands of people of all ages are faced with that very scenario. I was one of them. How a person faces it can mean the difference between a life of sorrow and a life rich with possibility. Among other mindsets, I had hope, and I made the decision to beat the odds and face my diagnosis of incurable cancer with a will to live.

Hope sustains people when they face some great emergency or some difficult situation in life. Others have seen, as I have, those who have been stricken with life-threatening illness and faced death. I looked it in the eye and chose life. I wanted to live. Regardless of the odds, I chose hope.

For many hope lives on a continuum that runs from total despair to optimal positivity. My hope was and is self-determined, and it impacted the way I received news from my medical providers. I believed my treatments were working, and most importantly I defined how I sought information and opportunities to expand my control over my own well-being.

I enjoyed John Denver's music and inspirational verses over his lifetime and during my younger days. I particularly liked to hear his voice at concerts and when skiing down the mountains of Utah, Colorado, Wyoming, or California. Yet another poem, a Sanskrit proverb, reinforces the John Denver melody "I Want to Live".

> *Look to this day for it is life,*
> *For yesterday is already a dream,*
> *And tomorrow is only a vision.*
> *But today, well lived, makes every yesterday*
> *A dream of happiness and every tomorrow, a vision of hope.*

There is an unspoken bond of understanding among cancer survivors, people with cancer, and their friends and families.

They share empathy, depression, anxiety about the future, and fear of suffering and/or dying. An individual's attitude toward his or her illness and, by extension, the way in which he or she portray it to others determines how friends, family, and colleagues react. Contact with other human beings stimulates hope.

The confrontation with mortality is a wake-up call that leads many individuals to reassess values and either to confirm or to change their way of life. Of all the ingredients of the will to live, none is more essential than hope. Hope means different things to different people. One person may hope for the fullest possible remaining life. Another may hope to live until a special holiday or a family event. Still another may simply hope to avoid suffering.

Doctors can contribute substantially to a patient's feelings of hope. When a patient asks, "How long have I got?" some physicians will respond, "Six months," "A year," or "Two years," and they quote clinical statistics for that person's disease. What these physicians are forgetting to mention is that statistics are averages compiled from survival data on a great number of individuals. My doctors at first indicated "three months" and then changed it to "a few weeks." As many cancer survivors demonstrate, it is impossible to predict any person's longevity. Prognostication regarding one's mortality is based primarily on data. The unknowns are the individual's attitude, will to live, and other internal and external traits.

For centuries doctors followed Hippocrates's injunction to hold out hope to patients even when it meant withholding the truth. However, that canon has been blasted apart by modern patients' demands for honesty and more involvement in their care. Now patients may be told more than they need or want to know. Yet they still also need and want hope.

When a doctor suggests that an exhausted patient try yet another grueling therapy in the hope that it may extend survival by weeks, the cost is also considerable—financially, physically, and emotionally. "We have to find a less toxic way to manage their hope," said Dr. Nicholas A. Christakis, an internist and Harvard professor who is writing a textbook about prognosis.

We hope that the cancer was caught early, that the doctor will get all the cancer when he or she does the surgery, and that the cancer hasn't spread. A consensus is emerging that all patients need hope and that doctors should offer it in some form.

Dr. Joseph Sacco, a palliative care specialist at Bronx-Lebanon Hospital Center, wrote in an e-mail for an article titled, "Doctors' Delicate Balance in Keeping Hope Alive," "We prognosticate because people ask us to and trust our judgment. They do not know the depth of our uncertainty or that no matter how good or experienced we are, we are often wrong."

Diane Behar, writing on the Internet site Cancer Supportive Care Programs, expressed herself concerning her cancer journey in "One Patient's Way of Coping" in this way:

> Somewhere inside the deepest part of me, my truest self hides out under cover, and tells me that all of this is temporary and that I must just wait out these drug-induced episodes. This kind voice, along with my unwavering faith in God, enables me to conquer and think somehow I will be able to see my way into the clearing. And so I go on.

An insight into her whole experience may be read on the Internet at http://www.cancersupportivecare.com/cope.html.

There is no medicine like hope
No incentive so great
And no tonic so powerful
As the expectation
Of something better tomorrow
—Orison Swett Marden, MD
Founder of *Success Magazine*

Optimism and Hope

Jerome Groopman, MD, author of *The Anatomy of Hope*, writes that sometimes very bad things happen to wonderful people. He explains that a positive attitude (optimism) is the thought that "everything is going to turn out for the best." He says hope, in contrast, doesn't make that same assumption. Rather, with a clear head and understanding of the facts and with due diligence, such as assessing the issues, challenges and obstacles, hope allows the person to move forward with increased understanding of the whole picture after one educates him or herself with information. Through such a process, the hopeful person will then seek out and pursue a plan, a realistic one that is intended to lead to an improved future.

With regard to the difference between hope and optimism, in his book, *Standing on the Promises*, Professor Lewis Smedes states it this way:

This is what makes hope different from optimism. Optimists live by evidence and their optimism dies when the hard data point to defeat. People of hope live by faith, and their hope lives on even after the life support of tangible evidence shuts itself off. People of hope dig into their faith and draw on it when the vital signs of reason grow faint. People of hope have to be people of faith.

127

Hope

What is this thing called hope? What goes on inside of us when we hope? Why do we need hope for our spirits the way we need food and water for our bodies? Why is hope as crucial to our lives as our sanity? How can we become more hopeful people? How can we keep on hoping when our fondest hopes crash on the rugged edges of tragedy?

Shortly after I had my first surgery on my head and into my skull, my longtime closest friend, Sam, shared with me a book. In it, Sam wrote this to me: "We can't see beyond today as God can, so He gives us the Gift of Hope for the journey, as an expression of His love for us."

True hope is not blind optimism. It sees reality and all the problems and challenges ahead as well as the potential for failure. With this hope, people find a hidden inner strength, the strength to brace themselves for the difficult road ahead, the strength to see clearly and make very smart decisions. "Keep hope alive" was not just rhetoric for me.

Real hope gives us a sense of energy and control, even in desperate circumstances. Instead of the question "Why me?" I was intent on further exploring "Why not me?"

In my cancer support community group one of our fellow participants was vocal about those who preached the power of hope. He strongly believed that hopelessness was just as important and that too much positivism was contrary to the well-being of many. At the center of his argument was the notion that false hope doesn't serve anyone very well, particularly those of us who have more advanced cancer, in which even the best success with treatment might mean a matter of weeks or perhaps an extra month or two of life. It clearly was a topic of considerable interest to all of us.

When I faced cancer, I wanted answers. I also wanted hope. And I wanted both at the same time.

The primary way to move through adversity is to maintain a strong, positive mental attitude regardless of the circumstances and the challenges that we face. In other words, it is important to have hope. One has to identify what questions need to be asked, whom one needs to see, what the options are, and how to move forward. "I cannot direct the wind, but I can adjust my sails," is a saying, and it is a pretty good philosophy for life.

The support and encouragement of family and friends in the presence of adversity make up one of the most important elements of hope. The uncomplicated, direct love and simple trust of two of our grandchildren, Evie and Adam, have been priceless to me.

I remember one time when my small grandson said to me, "Grandpa, I don't want you to die!"

I had picked him up after kindergarten. Intending to surprise him and help our daughter-in-law, Nichole, so that she could have some additional time for herself, I had arrived eager to see his face when I stood outside the schoolyard with the mothers who were there to pick up their children.

About fifteen mothers and I stood and waved as the children lined up and waved back. As each came through the gate from the schoolyard, a smile and greeting of some sort occurred, with excited children and happy mothers all embracing. Adam was one of those near the front of the line.

As Adam came out and saw me, he beamed, grabbed me, gave me a special hug, and took my hand. Then the fun began as we walked away from the schoolyard. Holding my hand tightly, Adam looked up at each mother nearby and announced with a loud voice to each one, "Hi, this is my grandpa. He picked me up. He is very sick. He has cancer. He is going to die soon!"

Let me just say that we moved along at a much faster pace than originally intended. Actually I dragged Adam as he kept on mouthing the words. As we approached the car, I tried to figure out what I was going to say. Finally when he and I were both buckled into the seat belts, I turned around to him and said that I appreciated his concern but that things were going a little better, even though I might not look like it.

With that, Adam unbuckled his seat belt, stood up in the backseat, gave me a big hug around my neck, and said those immortal words that almost brought tears to my eyes, "Grandpa, I don't want you to die. I love you."

Hope is the seed from which faith grows. Faith doesn't grow without hope.

My greatest hope is that we will find a cure for cancer of all types. Complete eradication of it from our planet is something I pray for almost every day—not just my cancer but everyone's. Notice how I have now personalized it as being *mine*. My hope is that this disease doesn't get to affect the lives of any more precious people.

The Role of the Mind in Hope

In our lives we usually cannot choose the mountains that face us, but we can choose the best paths on which to ascend them.

The mind has such power! It is evidenced by the people who walk on coals and have no ill effects. Such power can be used for improving the body's health and altering its responses. What is critical to the survival and recovery of cancer victims is the realization that they *do* have a choice in how they feel. They have the power to choose whether they are going to feel good or bad. The human body will react in ways that the mind tells it to, and there is plenty of scientific evidence to support this fact!

Keeping hope alive and encouraging others who might be discouraged, avoiding being consumed by hopelessness by removing pride, and letting others be a part of our lives can help us deal with the pain we are experiencing.

Research and Perspectives on Hope

An increasing number of studies are suggesting that a positive attitude can play a significant role in a cancer patient's reaction to treatment and recovery.

In his book *The Power of Hope: A Doctor's Perspective*, Dr. Howard Spiro explores how patients and caring doctors can help lessen suffering when illness occurs. He urges that physicians focus on their patients' feelings of pain and anxiety as well as on their physical symptoms.

Dr. Tone Rusteen and his health-care team undertook a study titled "The Importance of Hope as a Mediator of Psychological Distress and Life Satisfaction in a Community Sample of Cancer Patients." They pointed out that although hope is an important resource for cancer patients, few studies include it as an independent or dependent variable in quality-of-life research.

Yet another study with a focus on hope was undertaken in 2007 by Grace Chu-Hui-Lin Chi. Its title is "The Role of Hope in Patients with Cancer." The purpose of the study, which appeared in the March 2007 Oncology Nursing Forum, was to synthesize the literature, develop generalizations, and identify issues that should be evaluated in the future in regard to hope and patients with cancer.

Dr. Jerome Groopman's excellent book *The Anatomy of Hope: How People Prevail in the Face of Illness* cites evidence from well-controlled experiments. When challenged, patients' bodies perform differently based on their minds' expectations. Movingly he describes decades of being with patients as they faced probable death and details his journey as a physician learning to help them deal with it. He writes,

> Hope, unlike optimism, is rooted in unalloyed reality. ... Hope acknowledges the significant obstacles and deep pitfalls along the path. True hope has no room for delusion.
>
> Clear-eyed, hope gives us the courage to confront our circumstances and the capacity to surmount them. For all my patients, hope, true hope, has proved as important as any medication.

In his insightful book written more than thirty years ago, *The Biology of Hope*, the late Norman Cousins said about the role of patients in the partnership between the doctor and the patient,

> Any battle with serious illness involves two elements. One was represented by the ability of the physicians to make available to patients the best that medical science has to offer. The other element was represented by the ability of patients to summon all their physical and spiritual resources in fighting illness.

Observations Concerning Hope

Hope also implies dependence on forces outside ourselves. Hope has been an integral component of the healing and recovery process for centuries. Arlene Harder is founder and editor-in-chief of the websites Support4Change.com and ChildhoodAffirmations. com. She has been a licensed psychotherapist for more than twenty years, a cofounder of The Wellness Community-Foothills in Pasadena, California, and an author. In her article "The Nature and Complexity of Hope," she ably offers insights and observations from her experience with cancer patients and others as they deal with the issues around illness and hope for the future.

We may not know as much about the role of hope as we will in the future, but here are some things we do know now.

►**Hope exists within a realistic context of uncertainty**.

When we move ahead with plans for a vacation, we hope to enjoy ourselves, although we are clearly aware that potential obstacles like the weather and airline strikes are beyond our control. A person who has hope in the face of a life-threatening illness likewise moves forward with quiet confidence. For example, if the statistics for cancer patients indicate there is only a 10% probability of survival, they will approach life as though those figures can apply to them. Some are able to identify more strongly with the 10%, and others will believe themselves part of the 90%.

►**Hope is a crucial antidote to fear.**

The unknown that lies within a diagnosis of cancer and other serious illness raises many fears and anxieties. Unlike the person who denies the reality of the diagnosis in an effort to avoid having to deal openly with frightening and unsettling emotions, a person with hope realizes that the future may not turn out as he or she would like and, nevertheless, chooses to believe the future is somehow benevolent. Such a person focuses on potential rather than limitation.

►**The "meaning" and "purpose" of our lives are intertwined with hope.**

As Jeanne Achterberg of the Saybrook Institute in San Francisco has suggested, hope is the "enduring feeling that life makes sense." When life makes sense, it can be transcended in the sense that one can rise above it psychologically and not be emotionally defeated by it. It is possible that by taking such a position a person may actually live longer.

►**What is hoped for changes during the course of illness.**

The National Coalition for Cancer Survivorship calls this "the changing mosaic of hope." When symptoms force us to see the doctor for an examination, as we wait for the results we hope there won't be anything seriously wrong. After a diagnosis of serious illness, generally the first thing for which we hope is a complete cure. Later, after treatment, we may hope for an extended period of remission before the disease recurs or for control of symptoms for a long time. When the disease is in the advanced stage, there is still much to hope for: living to see a daughter graduate, energy to take a trip to some place we've always wanted to visit, a slow rate of deterioration, lessening of pain, having a peaceful, dignified death.

►**Action requires hope.**

In order to plan for the future, to research the latest medical advances, and to take part in decisions concerning treatment options, a person needs the ability to imagine that his or her efforts may be at least potentially successful.

►Hope permeates all dimensions of a person's life.

People with hope have a greater sense of energy. Most of the time their mood is more likely to be up than down, despite obstacles. Because they feel more confident, they ask more questions. They are also more persistent, and a busy, impatient doctor may not view them as "good" patients, while more passive, and less hopeful, patients may be.

►There are many sources of hope.

For some, hope comes from a belief that God cares for them. For others, hope arises from a belief that research can discover a cure. Others may believe their doctor knows best and put themselves in the hands of their medical team.

►Hope expects—and needs—reinforcement and external support.

While hope can exist in the absence of uniform agreement that a goal will be reached (in which case success may not need much hope because the probability of achieving it may almost be assured), maintaining hope in the face of total opposition is extremely difficult. That is why hopeful people are connected with other people and with the things they care about. They are thus able to draw strength from their families, their beliefs, their participation in what needs to be done toward reaching their goals, and in the medical procedure they choose. This is why it is important that family and friends understand their role in supporting the patient who wants to hope for the best.

What Is Hope?

Any choice that moves your inner thoughts toward hope and possibility can make you feel happier and physically stronger.

Hope sustains people when they are faced with emergencies or when critical situations occur. Marty, though afflicted by a severe stroke impacting her mind, eyesight, and her right side, has been determined to be able to walk and use her arms and legs in a manner that will be a new normal for her. Her perseverance, determination, hope, and faith have made her more successful than anyone could have imagined at the time this traumatic event occurred.

"Hope" is the thing with feathers—
That perches in the soul—
And sings the tune without the words—
And never stops—at all—

And sweetest—in the Gale—is heard—
And sore must be the storm—
That could abash the little Bird
That kept so many warm—

I've heard it in the chillest land—
And on the strangest sea—
Yet never in Extremity,
It asked a crumb - of me.

—Emily Dickinson
American poet

In *The Long Walk to Freedom*, Nelson Mandela draws attention to the importance of hope. He had to wait in prison for twenty-seven years before his hope of a new South Africa could be achieved. As the day of his freedom drew close, his only daughter was allowed to come and see him. When she came, she carried with her the grandchild Mandela had never seen. She had waited to name the girl until her grandfather could give her a name. "I don't think a man was ever happier to hold a baby than I was that day," he wrote in his memoirs. Mandela named her Zaziwe, an African word for hope. He called her Hope, he said, because "during all my years in prison hope never left me—and now it never would."

Although worry and fear are almost automatic when one is dealing with cancer, there are personal decisions to be made. Some people tell cancer sufferers to give it up, to let hope die and let worry die with it. And they have us almost convinced. However, because of hope, many choose to keep on pursuing the avenues open to us.

Although we cannot control the future, the attitude we choose toward tomorrow affects life today. I am engaged in the adventure of increasing my conscious contact with my God through prayer and the fellowship of others who are also so engaged. My hope is founded in what I already feel in my life.

With hope, nothing is so overwhelming that we can't move forward, and nothing we really need will be beyond our grasp.

Miles Strodel, my high school coach, teacher, mentor, nurturer, confidant, and friend, wrote to me when I arrived at my small college in the Midwest. I was a transplanted Bostonian amidst the cornfields and wide-open spaces of Indiana. In addition to words of encouragement and an invitation to call on him and his wife, Grace—(I refer to this lovely woman as Amazing Grace and Mom as she took me under her wing in the earliest formative days)—at any time, he provided me with my life's underpinnings, particularly as I later dealt with the realities of my cancer diagnoses and treatment regimens.

To live with hope is a reflection on our attitude and perspective of life. To rebuild our foundation of hope, we need the courage to live. How we live and what we do with our lives is our choice and can be within our control subject to fate and good fortune. Yet when God and cancer meet, hope cannot be far away.

> May the God of hope fill you with all joy and peace as
> you trust in Him, so that you may overflow with hope.
> —Romans 15:13 NIV

Not Somehow but Triumphantly

This dynamic maxim encapsulates my ongoing journey with cancer since 1997. As I wrote this book, progressively I felt fine. I also know what the possibilities are. Once diagnosed with only a few weeks to live, I was reminded that someone once said that the ultimate statistic is that one person in one will die. We all know that our turn will come. The sands of time will run out. In that sense, we all face illnesses that will claim our lives, even if we are currently in good health and even if it comes very suddenly.

Knowing now that I was very ill helped me focus on life's brevity sooner than I wanted to think about it.

The Bible says that human life is like a breath or a shadow. Healthy people can easily ignore that reality.

Strangely facing the fact of death can be—and in my case has been—a big advantage and led to personal blessings once the initial shock of diagnosis had passed. It is also true for those seeing a loved one suffer serious illness.

From the outset of my diagnosis, I had an uncommon philosophy based in part on the scripture, "We also exult in our tribulations; knowing that tribulation brings about perseverance" (Romans 5:3 NASB).

Another word for perseverance is fortitude—the end result of pressure.

Fortitude is the God-given ability to face the storms of life head-on and come out not somehow ... but triumphantly.

"In the world you have tribulation," Jesus said, "but be of good cheer, I have overcome the world" (John 16:33). I love the title of the book by Dr. V. Raymond Edman, a former president of Wheaton College, and shared with me by my high school coach and his wife, Miles and Grace Strodel. It so gloriously sums up what a Christian's attitude should be in the midst of difficult times. Do you know what it is? "Not somehow but triumphantly." Not just getting through it somehow but triumphantly.

The Power of Faith

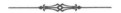

Faith is the confident assurance that what we hope for is going
to happen. It is the evidence of things we cannot yet see.
—Hebrews 11:1 NLT

As my faith became stronger, I was reminded that a little faith
is all that I needed. The Bible says that the smallest amount of
faith, no more than a mustard seed, is sufficient. God takes it
from there.

I came to the realization that I wake up every day filled
with confidence, enthusiasm, and gratitude for my blessings
as a result of my journey with cancer. I see that some of my
troubling moments were really blessings in disguise. Or to say it
in a different way, if I have breath in the morning, I have purpose.
I am prepared to live life.

Faith in the context of my cancer equals belief and certainty
that I can achieve my goal of doing whatever it takes to beat the
cancer that I have. This faith strengthens my motivation to act
and helps me maintain the positive attitude necessary for success.
My faith is important to me, but alone it is not enough for success.
I also need willpower, discipline, and persistence. I need to take
positive action in dealing with my cancer to demonstrate that the
words regarding "my faith is strong" is my reality.

I try in my daily efforts to take it a day at a time or moment by moment to do the right thing and, more importantly, to be that person who allows my commitments, determination, and focus to contribute to winning this battle.

"Came to believe" is a magical phrase for many who have awakened or reawakened to something beyond their immediate control. And what did I come to believe? That power—my faith and my God—greater than myself could restore and revitalize me. It is a basic tenet of my attitude in facing the unknown with cancer and in all aspects of my life. "Coming to believe" isn't usually a sudden happening but a gradual change. As I made an effort to strengthen my faith—a lesson learned in dealing with my wife's stroke as well as my own journey with cancer—I found it makes my life work.

Personally I came to believe that my God never gave me more than I could handle. In 1 Corinthians 10, Paul writes, "God is faithful; he will not let you be tempted beyond what you can bear. But when you are tempted, he will also provide a way out so that you can stand up under it."

Cancer is a disruptive, life-altering experience for most patients and their families. In the face of grueling treatments, unruly symptoms, and uncertainty about the future, many express the important role personal faith and spirituality play in helping them cope. Faith is a powerful force that all of humanity has yet to embrace. Many people have read the previous biblical verse and yet have not incorporated the concept into their lives. Many people live below their God-given potentials because they have not had faith in themselves and all that Scripture has taught.

For many people achieving goals and living successful lives, a faith in God is a secret. The scriptures have made many promises, but when challenges arise, these promises are frequently forgotten. Obstacles will come up, but the depth of faith determines people's strength in handling them. People with faith are more likely to

141

handle stresses like doubt, fear, insecurity, etc., as they occur. If not for faith, some technological advancements would have been impossible. Following the concepts of dreams and faith, achievements such as travel to outer space become a reality. Even those who have the most faith expect challenges but move through these impediments with more strength.

Addressing a perspective on the importance of one's faith, Dr. Herbert Benson of Harvard University had this to say: "Faith is often an invisible force which carries great healing power ... It is a supremely potent belief."

Through my journey I have been reminded multiple times of the book by Thomas Hardy, *Far from the Madding Crowd*. Its focus was on the ever-increasing industrialization and commercialization of life. Hardy discussed a significant dilemma. Even when surrounded with so much activity and hordes of people, how was it possible to feel so alone? Where do people seek comfort and inner peace?

Embracing One's Faith

Remez Sasson, a teacher and writer on positive thinking, creative visualization, motivation, self-improvement, peace of mind, and spiritual growth, commented in her book *Visualize and Achieve*,

> The power of faith and belief is real power. Believing that you can attain your goal is of great importance for its achievement. Without faith, there will be doubts and disbelief, which lead to non-doing and to non-achievement. Faith draws and attracts what you want into your life, whereas doubts, worries and disbelief push them away.

Religious Faith and Faith in Ourselves

The word *faith* can be found a total of 304 times in the New Testament of the King James Version of the Holy Bible according to Project Gutenberg. Yet when I first considered whether or not there was any difference between religious faith and having faith in myself, I explored what others—not philosophers or theologians but more or less the people on the street—offered in response to the question, "Are there differences or similarities between religious faith and faith in ourselves?"

Since there seemed to be some disagreement as to the similarities and differences between religious faith and faith in ourselves as concepts, as a reality check I decided to investigate what faith is from a theological perspective.

Michael Fackerell, a theologian in Australia, has provided some ideas on the subject in his Christian Faith.com blog (http://www.christian-faith.com/faith-in-god/) titled, "Faith in God." He has described faith in terms that have helped me in my journey with cancer.

> In the general sense of the word, to have faith is to believe in something or someone, to fully trust, to be so confident that you base your actions on what you believe. To have faith is to be fully convinced of the truthfulness and reliability of that in which you believe.

He goes on to indicate that faith is a spiritual substance, a response to God's Word, and a spiritual force. Integral to one's faith is not only embracing hope but also acting in ways that reflect one's faith and call to action. Said another way, if one is to live in faith, it means that we need to do and say what we believe is right.

Life should be the process of making progress. We learn by doing, not just by thinking. We can make forward steps more easily when we ask our God to share the journey, but we have to put one foot in front of the other. That usually leads in the right direction.

Faith has a way of bringing us into a certain sense of understanding that we are sustained by a loving, friendly, powerful God. That is the gift of faith. You can say, "I am sustained by the Lord. What would I do—where would I be without by faith?" Many do not have the same sense, and it's a terrible thing because their lives are deprived of the benefits that come from faith—the empowerment, the peace, and all the rest.

Walk the Walk

> Every life is a profession of faith, and exercises
> an inevitable and silent influence.
> —Henri Frederic Amiel
> Swiss philosopher, poet, and critic

What an individual does or doesn't believe shows, and the intensity of beliefs will have a positive or negative impact on other people. Each individual has control over his or her attitude. The ability to change our minds and moods is one of the greatest powers for good or evil we have.

In the face of a serious illness, faith can offer the comfort that comes from connecting with a greater power. Though there is no evidence that spirituality alone can cure cancer or other diseases, a study from the American Cancer Society shows that faith can reduce stress, loneliness, pain, and anxiety, and give some people with health challenges peace of mind and the will to live.

I was reminded each day that faith can be nurtured. One can learn how to pray. It is neither magic nor necessarily the pathway to instant miracles. My experience reminded me how incredibly powerful my faith was, as it helped to provide inner peace, hope, and emotional balance.

Why do prayer and faith seem to improve health? Experts think the overall feelings of community and belonging that the faithful have go a long way toward decreasing the stress that illness and disability can bring. Rather than having to go it alone, they can place their problems in other hands. It is very similar to the positive effect support groups have. Most twelve-step programs rely significantly on faith to support those attempting to overcome addiction.

Religion may not be for everyone, but if a person is open and willing to do what it takes to improve his or her health, he or she may want to check out a house of worship. Said person won't be alone.

Faith can be nurtured. Everyone can learn how to pray. It is neither magic nor the pathway to instant miracles, yet for some it is incredibly powerful and can provide inner peace, hope, and emotional balance. It is important to know that despite the connections people share with others, there is something else, God, to whom they can turn to find a measure of peace.

My second experimental phase-one clinical trial was intended to reduce the tumors in my spleen and elsewhere in my body. The trial was to run for between two and two and a half years. After almost six months, during which I was being monitored closely, I came to realize that what was occurring was contrary to the intended outcome. I looked at the laboratory results, CT and PET scans, the MRI on my brain, and the ongoing evaluation of the extent to which the infusions were working. Even with the oncologists and their staff monitoring me closely and encouraging me, I knew my body was not responding as I had hoped or as the oncologists had thought I might.

In the eighth month I had the routine consultation and monitoring procedure. When I met with my oncologist, I was informed I would no longer be in the trial as my tumors were growing at a more pronounced rate. During the past few trial cycles, they had been slowly growing at a 1 percent rate for every six-week cycle. In the past six weeks, however, they had grown almost 5 percent larger and had grown 25 percent larger than the baseline size from when I'd begun the trial.

How did I react? With fear or with depression? On the contrary, I had a peace within me and calmly said to my oncologist, "I knew it already. Thank you for telling me. Now what is Plan C, and what options are available to me?"

The stronger our spiritual connection, the less we will be held back by our fears and self-doubts. If we can call upon a trusted guide, we'll never lack support.

Eternal truths are always fresh. That is why so many people treasure a daily visit with a spiritual guide through meditation. Each day we can refresh our spirits with the help of such a guide. Meditation is a process of simplifying, emptying out, and concentrating our minds so that we can be open to a spiritual experience. This has worked for me.

A Transformative Journey

Surveys show that 90 percent of American adults believe in God. Many feel faith is one of the most important forces in their lives. Faith can give people the strength to cope with whatever happens in life. Yet no matter the strength of a person's faith, it is not unusual for it to be shaken by a cancer diagnosis. Feelings of punishment or abandonment by God are not uncommon. In my case, it wasn't so much about God and punishment or prayers being answered or not. It was more along the lines of "What do I truly believe?" and "Is my faith strong enough?" as well as "Who am I as a person?"

Faith is an amazing power. I have found that in my life, my faith has become a very powerful means for fulfillment. As I gained strength in my faith, there was a greater momentum toward my goal of beating cancer. Some amazing transformations in my daily life have occurred.

We reconnected with Jean and her husband, Vin, who lived on the East Coast. My life was made richer and more whole because of this friendship. Jean was a schoolteacher and educational consultant, and she had been a college faculty member. Vin had been a pastor to an inner-city church in the New England area, had served as a college president for more than a decade, and had been the director of a Christian counseling center in Connecticut. They have two daughters. Marty and I developed a warm though long-distance friendship. During the early days of the evolving friendship, none of us anticipated we would be drawn together even closer by a mutual bonding agent—cancer.

Vin was diagnosed with advanced colon cancer in 2002. Monitoring his regimen of surgery and chemotherapy, meeting with some of the best medical experts in the country, and also trying to maintain his counseling practice took its toll on his energy. Yet he was almost always uplifting when we talked either via telephone, in person, or via e-mail.

Vin's cancer spread to other organs, and his condition worsened. He was a fighter. With new therapies, his oncologists were actively engaged in research and trying to help Vin. Jean was at his side as caregiver and as support for his frequent hospitalizations, surgeries, radiation treatments, and a number of emergency runs to the hospital. Despite the challenges Vin faced early on in his journey with cancer, he retained a positive, upbeat outlook and an attitude that lifted those who cared for him and loved him very much.

In our exchanges after I was diagnosed with advanced melanoma in 2005, Vin would write, "Keep hope alive! It's the only thing powerful enough to pull us forward when circumstances would otherwise capture us and hold us back."

On another occasion Vin responded to my progress in dealing with my own journey. "Thanks for your always timely and encouraging thoughts. One of my clients, a mother of a teenager who is borderline with a sister who struggles with mental illness told me this morning that she often hears from skeptical friends who wonder how she can believe in God when she has had so much suffering in her own life. She looked at me and with a great deal of passion said, 'How could I survive if I didn't believe in Him?' She has it right."

In March of 2006, Marty and I flew to Florida to spend a week with Jean and Vin. It was evident that Vin was in a lot of pain; however, he didn't say anything, and he slept a lot on most days. We did some things together. When Vin couldn't go someplace where we all had intended to go, he told Jean to go along. He told her that he would be fine. We soon left for California after we were assured that he was stable. After that visit we kept in touch and communicated frequently.

I thought it important to put in writing to Jean and Vin some of my thoughts on what was going on in both of our lives. Over the years Vin was a beacon of light and hope for those whose lives he touched. People continued to be uplifted by him because of his testimony, his life, and how he helped others. They listened to his excellent advice and counsel and were moved to action by his caring and supportive ways. "Others still need you," I wrote to Vin, "as an inspiration, as a sage, and as being a seasoned veteran of the journey. You have not faded away, nor will people allow you to do that. Rather, as your own journey continues you remain steadfast in your testimony, helping others, caring for so many others, and with the knowledge, hopefully, that God is not ready to call you home but rather is using you as a positive role model for many others."

In September of 2006, Vin had to be rushed to the hospital for emergency surgery. Jean and their daughters wrote,

> His journey has been long and ongoing. I have hesitated to send another email telling you all of this news and yet at the same time was anxious to share our concerns for this new development. We as a family are most blessed with the caring and prayerful people who have seen us through so much the last 4 years. We could not have made it without you!

Later in the month Jean wrote again about Vin's continuing fighting spirit as well as ongoing treatments. "Pray for continued strength, hope, peace, and calm for Vin. His very close friends have been an awesome support to us since his emergency surgery three weeks ago."

It was clear Vin and his family had not given up. Like Vin, they had hope and determination, and through this entire journey they continued to serve others while they also served themselves. The impact this had on any who knew what they were going through was significant.

While Vin was undergoing his treatments and interventions, I was also having surgeries. We shared some common experiences on the surgical front as well as the subsequent experiences with our medical teams. How fortunate we both were to have loving families, excellent medical attention, and the strength that came from our faith.

In October, Jean wrote an update on Vin and said that he was strong enough, according to his medical team, to undergo yet another surgery to address the cancer now in his lungs and elsewhere. In her most caring and thoughtful way in reaching out to others, Jean included this in her note to us and several others: "Our continued thanks for all the love, concern and prayers you have continued to support us with through these many, many surgeries. We are blessed beyond measure with our extended families and friends."

In late October, Vin sent me a note in response to one of my notes to him. Here again, like Jean, he touched Marty and me in a special way.

> Please know how much the whisper you spoke on our behalf is heard clear across the miles and has touched us once again in a special way. We continue to lift you up to the One who is Higher than all. Love and blessing again to you and Marty.

Jean and Vin wrote to Marty and me in late November. Vin was still in the hospital, this time for eight weeks. Once again their message was clear.

> Thank you for letting us share in the blessing it [the book *Standing on the Promises*] was for you during these days we all seem to be facing. We have a lot of unknowns but knowing the one who holds our futures with love, care and understanding of the struggles we find ourselves in. It is a peaceful feeling to know He *is* our constant guide, support, and only security.

Some more insights from Vin arrived a few days later as he was up and about and back in his counseling center, meeting with clients. He thanked me again for sharing the book with him and made the following pertinent observations:

Hope is ultimately the only thing we have to keep us from getting stuck in Now and likewise is the only thing powerful enough to keep pulling us forward—as the apostle Paul would say, right into eternity. Since hope is one of the easiest things to let go of in the midst of our struggles, I appreciated the reminders of its importance in our daily lives—so thanks for thinking of us and sending the book our way.

A little less than a month later on December 24, 2006, Jean, in reminding us of the great *gift* that is reflected in our Christmas celebration, included in her note a reminder of things that are always on our mind as we move forward on our own journey.

We treasure what you have meant to us during this entire journey. Vin remains in a rehab/hospice facility where he has been given outstanding care. For this we are so grateful. He is growing weaker each day. We covet your prayers for his peace and comfort in these last days.

The Reverend Vincent E. Taber, seventy, died peacefully after a courageous battle with cancer on January 2, 2007. Jean has remained a dear friend, and Marty and I have visited with her in California as well as on Cape Cod. I am reminded of a prayer that someone shared with me that seems appropriate at this time … or anytime.

O God, the strength of those who labor
and the rest of the weary,
grant us when we are tired with our work to be
recreated by your Spirit;
that being renewed for the service of your kingdom,

151

we may serve you gladly in freshness
of body and mind; through Jesus Christ our Lord.
Amen.

God's way is ours. He won't be rushed; all will happen in good time. The future is in God's hands. Our own special days will come. One thing is certain: with trust in God's love—and His amazing grace—all future days will be good.

A second transforming experience for me occurred in June 2010. A person unknown to me at the time had taken the liberty of sending out a message to many people from my undergraduate college, Taylor University, a small Christian liberal arts institution of higher learning in Indiana. The message indicated that I had cancer. She indicated I had asked for the prayers of people receiving this information. As a private person who had not communicated with fellow alumni in the fifty years since graduation, I was really, really upset. I felt my privacy had been violated. To say that I was unhappy would be a gross understatement.

After I fussed and fumed over the breach of what I considered normal etiquette and respect for others, I talked with my wife. Should I send a blistering letter to the person who'd sent it out, call and give a piece of my mind, or take the high road and let it go? We decided that I should let it go. It turned out that the communication resulted in a significant and important transformation in my life as it relates to my faith.

A couple who received the communication, George and Jan Glass, were friends of mine in college. I had not had any interaction with either of them for more than fifty years. Jan had been a teacher, school counselor, and high school guidance counselor. A standout in college as a student and in cocurricular activities, she'd carried her strengths to her family, church, and community. Jan was recognized as teacher of the year in Indiana. George had been an outstanding athlete in high school and college. He'd later coached high school athletics, gone on to be a college coach of track and field, and then returned to our alma mater to coach cross country before he became the athletic director at our alma mater. Recognized nationally and internationally for his contributions to athletics and student athletes, George, like Jan, was a sought-after public speaker. He also volunteered his time in their church and in multiple venues in his community. They had four children and several grandchildren, all of them very successful in all that they were doing in education, careers, and family life.

There in my in-box was a message from Jan a few weeks later. In it she expressed concern about my illness and said she and George had been praying for me since they'd received the e-mail. She also went on to ask a question or two regarding the fiftieth golden anniversary class reunion and homecoming event for my graduating class. I answered the questions and offered to be helpful. In turn, she asked if I could help her. In fact, would I be willing to be cochair of the reunion committee? She had set the bait out and hooked me easily. However, I told her about feeling betrayed and violated by the letter that had been distributed without my knowledge or permission. Though I certainly believed in prayer and its power, I was a private person. I also told Jan that I didn't know how much help I could be, but I would do things when I was strong enough and would let her know if I was going to be able to do something or not. With that understanding, we agreed to be a team, have fun, move forward, and see what we could accomplish.

Jan understood the ground rules I had set for the both of us. More importantly she explained who the person who had revealed my cancer was and indicated that I should "get over it" and have some joy. I agreed, and so I began a long-distance cochairpersonship with Jan in Indiana and me in California. And did we have fun!

Through this partnership Jan and I also shared views on faith and spiritual matters. She and her husband George would lift my spirits, embrace me in my challenges, share their caring and love for me, and share many powerful truths for personal living. During the weeks and months of reunion planning, I was undergoing chemotherapy as well as the indignities of enduring scans, brain MRIs, blood draws, EKGs, and other tests along with a few other pokes and pinches that had become routine. All had side effects.

As Jan and I were assisted by a larger golden anniversary reunion committee in planning our fiftieth, Jan thought that a face-to-face committee meeting on the campus of Taylor University in Upland, Indiana, would be an important reality check of what needed to be accomplished. It was an opportunity to meet with campus staff to help them understand what all needed to be done. A meeting date was established. The majority of the committee was able to attend. Jan and George knew, as did Nelson Rediger and Delilah Earls from the Taylor staff, that I was undergoing treatments and wasn't certain that I would be able to travel to attend the meeting.

I was determined to attend the get-together. A few days before the scheduled date, I informed Jan that I was going to attend no matter what it took. We agreed that she and George would not tell anyone in case I wasn't able to travel, as I was having a chemotherapy treatment the day before my intended departure. I had a plane ticket to fly to Fort Wayne. Jan and George had invited me to stay with them and travel with them to and from the campus in Upland. When the day came, Marty dropped me off at Los Angeles airport, and I departed for Fort Wayne, Indiana.

Upon arrival I was able to recognize my two friends. Even with more than fifty years behind us, I could have picked them both out in Times Square. They looked terrific, and we all embraced with big hugs for a long time. Then we were off to their lovely home and the next day to Taylor University. (The airline had lost my luggage, so I had to borrow some clothes from George.)

My brief presence on the campus was one I will never forget. It was *my* homecoming in a way. I very much enjoyed being on Taylor's campus after many years. I believe it was only the second time I had been on the campus since I'd graduated. In a way I felt like the prodigal son returning to a place that once was his home. Though I had no expectations, my presentiment of my transformation began about a half hour before arrival on the campus with Jan and George.

I had followed with considerable interest the story of the tragic accident that had taken place a few miles away from the campus on April 26, 2006. Many have forgotten about it with the passage of time, although the tragedy was covered nationally on broadcasts all over the country and the world and struck a nerve in many people.

On that day a tractor-trailer driver fell asleep at the wheel, crossed over the median of a multilane interstate highway just outside of Marion, Indiana, and hit a southbound van carrying six Taylor students and a staff member returning from the Fort Wayne area. Only one student survived, and there was a case of mistaken identity regarding the lone survivor.

George and Jan pointed out to me the specific site as we traveled from their Fort Wayne home to the Upland campus. It was marked by several crosses along the side of the highway. I began to *feel* mentally and physically that I was being prepared for my campus homecoming. (I wiped away a few tears as well.) A personal and *spiritual* uplifting experience was unfolding.

Most people would say they know what homecoming means, but when they're pressed to identify its origins and purpose, their stories often become a little fuzzy. My return to the campus before the actual homecoming and reunion in October was a gift that unfolded throughout the day, beginning with George and Jan and causing many emotional connections as each *gift* was received and opened.

I really was overwhelmed by the comments each member of the committee made to me. I had not had any contact with most of them for fifty years or more. The very kind words spoken to me touched me deeply. In fact, I didn't quite know how to respond to the kindness and caring that was expressed in so many ways. All I could say was, "Thank you," from my heart.

After the committee meeting George was kind enough to take me on a trip around the campus to see the new buildings, current construction, and the changes that had occurred there. My memory of the grounds and facilities from back in 1956 was not of a campus but more of an array of buildings—not many— around a gym where I hung out quite a lot. What a change! What a transformation! What a beautiful use of space and architectural cohesiveness!

I made the connection of the crosses on the highway with the Taylor University Memorial Prayer Chapel. Standing as a "testimony and commitment of Taylor University, her students, faculty, staff, alumni, parents and friends to prayer," for me it provided a strong and central sense of place, as it reinforces the historic faith and life of this historic institution and the dedication of the Taylor family. I was moved deeply into my very being, my soul.

As others may know from their own journeys, when you are faced with life and death, when you are faced with trying to learn who you really are and what your true character is, you often learn a lot in terms of your priorities and what is important.

To me, a *sense of place* is making connections between the past and the present, between the events and places that are a distinctive part of who I am. It also means an environment that embodies its institutional culture, its values, and its purpose.

Each of us carries within ourselves a postage stamp of native soil. It is the memory of this place that nurtures us with identity and special strength, that provides what the Bible terms "the peace that passeth understanding." And it is to this place that each of us goes at various times in our lives as we move forward to find the deepest identity of self.

As we look not only at ourselves but also at our nation today, we see how memory and sense of place shape each of us. The Memorial Prayer Chapel became very special to me. In its silence and peaceful setting, the stories of students and staff that have gone to be with our Lord became very special to me. The chapel, through its setting on campus, its architecture, and its historic roots, spoke to my heart and reached deep into my soul.

I found myself reconnecting to myself and to, as Phillip Brooks calls them, "the great truths that we believe, the broad and general consecrations of our lives which we have made, the large objects of our desire, the great hopes and impulses that keep us at our work."

What have I learned from all this? That the early lessons are where the deepest truth is found. I left Taylor in 1960, and like a wanderer in Greek mythology, my travels brought me back to the place where I began my journey.

By returning to Taylor, in many ways I cut against the grain. We Americans are often taught to devalue the places we come from. We are taught to abandon old worlds. We are taught that to achieve success and make a mark in society, we must separate ourselves from our roots. Taylor believes that these places, memories, and values are essential to life and should not be abandoned in the name of progress.

The Memorial Prayer Chapel does not balkanize us by region or by caste, class, or gender. It bonds us as members of the Taylor family. It is a spiritual oasis on a campus where educational opportunity has been present for generations of students and faculty but also where prayer and commitment are integral to one's life journey. George and I stayed there for a long time. I was moved to tears by the loss of lives and the families that were all affected, as well as by the design and architecture that let one know this is a holy place, a place of serenity, peace, love, and joy.

Most important for me was the gratitude I had for being able to be back home in Indiana and have the spiritual affirmation and inner peacefulness I'd experienced on the campus in my youth. I was with people who embraced me with their unconditional love and their prayerful support for the future. That was very special for me. I felt a sense of connection and peace. It was beautiful.

As much as I had enjoyed and valued my Taylor experience as an undergraduate, I had wanted to leave it behind. The irony was that I couldn't wait to get out of there back then. I wanted a bigger universe. I was ready to fly. Now I had gone back to the place I'd wanted to leave behind. My return journey to Taylor with Jan and George and visiting there with Kathy, Bob, Carol, Jim, Roger, and many others turned out to be a journey home.

My time with Jan and George wasn't over yet. A couple of days later after we had spent hours just enjoying one another's company, they took me to their church in Fort Wayne. It was a lovely church—large, joyful, and full of His flock on that Sunday morning. Once again I sensed that God works in wondrous ways, and His amazing grace continues to be with me.

During the church service a video was shown of a church member, a young woman. With her husband they had two children. She was dealing with advanced cancer. The video was inspiring because of the progress she had made despite the doubtful prognosis for survival. The young woman thanked members of the church for their prayers and spoke of the power of prayer in helping the doctors and nurses as well as herself to deal with her treatment.

After the pastor finished his sermon and prayer, we all began to file out of our seats. As George and I slowly walked up the aisle toward an exit door, we both turned around to see Jan talking to the pastor. She was beckoning George and me to come back down toward the pulpit and stage.

Jan introduced me to her pastor, and he said that he understood from Jan that I was dealing with cancer. We spoke for a few minutes, and then he asked if he could pray for me. I responded in the affirmative. We all formed a circle, and each of us had our arms around one another, bowed our heads, and closed our eyes, and then the pastor began to pray … for me. At that moment I felt a kinship and a sense that someone else's arms were around my shoulders.

The auditorium was silent. I opened my eyes and glanced at the people in the auditorium. The social gatherings and low voices in the background had halted. I felt, real or imagined, that all of the energy in that auditorium was focused on me.

The pastor's words were thoughtful, helpful, personal, and uplifting. When he finished his prayer, I felt that I could fly with the eagles, as I had been lifted up by His presence and had an experience unlike any I'd ever had before. It was beautiful, peaceful, serene, and joyful.

On the way to Jan and George's home and then later when they took me to the airport to head back to Los Angeles, I felt blessed and had an inner peace that greatly surpassed my understanding.

Observations

> Faith never knows where it is being led, but it
> loves and knows the One who is leading.
> —Oswald Chambers
> Scottish theologian

One's faith and the belief in God provide solid, enduring strength to carry one through a cancer journey. Faith is believing in possibilities. It is the ability to carry on with our decisions to advance and cooperate with the interventions and treatment, even though we feel discouraged or tired. It is staying active in our relationships, even when we receive little in return or when our friends aren't able to respond.

If there was no doubt, there would be no need for faith. Faith is temporarily putting our doubts on the shelf and working toward our goals of beating the cancer through any means possible and believing that one can be not a statistic but a miracle. Faith is trusting that help and support will be there for us, even though they're not in view. It is looking at a map and choosing a new destination, getting on the path to go there, and trusting the marks on the map symbolize a real place we will find.

Faith is commitment to the moment, commitment to putting one foot in front of the other, to getting up in the morning and making breakfast. The day will bring what the day will bring. There will be things in our lives that seem unsure or doubtful. We cannot know what the outcome will be. Sometimes faith is simply a matter of continuing with our journey in the midst of doubt. What we can do is be faithful just one more day. Faith can and will grow. Faith is based on experience, the experience we gain with each small act and the competence that grows in us as a result of those acts.

Faith can also grow as a result of the trust we build with others as we work with them for mutual goals. Most importantly our faith grows as our relationship with our spiritual being, our God, and our mentor increases. Napoleon Hill, one of America's foremost success and motivational authors, said, "What the mind of man can conceive and believe, it can achieve." Faith is imperative if you are going to achieve your dreams, vision, and peace of mind. When following your dreams, I suggest you embrace this advice by the well-known New York writer and editor Dorothea Brande: "Act as if it is impossible to fail! And you will never experience failure, no matter what comes your way."

Here's to our success this year ... and always.

Addendum
Prostate Cancer

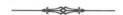

Cancer is a word, not a sentence.
—John Diamond
British broadcaster and journalist
who passed away from cancer in March 2001

Even though the primary focus of this book is on my experience with metastasized melanoma cancer, I would be remiss if I didn't draw brief attention to my prostate cancer. While I was dealing with the melanoma, I was diagnosed with prostate cancer. Though it was independent of my ongoing melanoma treatments, it had to be dealt with in a timely manner.

Through the miracles of modern medicine, today prostate disease is well-defined and is no longer necessarily considered a death sentence. Although prostate disease can be cured, late detection and delayed treatment can have grave consequences.

Why Is Prostate Cancer Important?

Other than skin cancer, prostate cancer is the most commonly diagnosed cancer in men. In fact, it is estimated that more than 230,000 men will be diagnosed with prostate cancer this year alone. According to the Centers for Disease Control and Prevention (CDC), after lung cancer, prostate cancer is the leading cause of cancer death among American men. The good news, however, is that the current survival rate is 97 percent. On average, an American man has a 30 percent risk of having prostate cancer in his lifetime but only a 3 percent risk of dying of the disease.

Also, among all racial and ethnic groups, prostate cancer death rates are declining. Perhaps the most encouraging prostate cancer statistic is that more men die *with* prostate cancer than *from* prostate cancer. The reason could be twofold. Prostate cancer typically affects men older than sixty-five, and it is often a slowly progressing disease.

The estimated lifetime risk of being diagnosed with the disease is 17.6 percent for Caucasians and 20.6 percent for African Americans. The lifetime risk of death from prostate cancer similarly is 2.8 percent and 4.7 percent respectively. As reflected in these numbers, prostate cancer is likely to impact the lives of a significant portion of men who are alive today.

Understanding Prostate Cancer

The prostate is part of a man's reproductive system. It is located in front of the rectum and under the bladder. It surrounds the urethra, the tube through which urine flows. A healthy prostate is about the size of a walnut. The prostate makes part of seminal fluid. During ejaculation seminal fluid helps carry sperm out of the man's body as part of semen. Male hormones (androgens) make the prostate grow. The testicles are the main source of male hormones, including testosterone. The adrenal gland also makes testosterone, but in small amounts. If the prostate grows too large, it squeezes the urethra. This may slow or stop the flow of urine from the bladder to the penis.

When prostate cancer spreads, cancer is often found in nearby lymph nodes, other lymph nodes, the bones, and/or other organs. When cancer spreads from its original place to another part of the body, the new tumor has the same kind of abnormal cells and the same name as the primary tumor. For example, if prostate cancer spreads to bones, the cancer cells in the bones are actually prostate cancer cells. The disease is metastatic prostate cancer, not bone cancer. For that reason, it is treated as prostate cancer, not bone cancer. Doctors call the new tumor *distant* or *metastatic* disease.

Risk Factors for Prostate Cancer in the United States

Age: Age is an important risk factor for prostate cancer. Prostate cancer is rarely seen in men younger than forty, but the chance of getting it goes up sharply as men get older. The chart below shows the probability of being diagnosed with prostate cancer for different age groups based on the National Cancer Institute's (NCI) "Cancer Risk: Understanding the puzzle."

Age Range	Probability of Prostate Cancer Diagnosis
Under Age 40	1 in 19,299

Ages 40 through 59	1 in 45
Ages 60 through 79	1 in 7

Race: Data from the NCI also indicates that African American men are at highest risk of prostate cancer. It tends to start at a younger age and grows faster than in men of other races. After African American men, it is most common among white men followed by Hispanic and Native American men. Asian-American men have the lowest rates of prostate cancer.

Family history: A man's risk of prostate cancer is higher than average if his father or brother had the disease. Prostate cancer risk also appears to be slightly higher for men whose mothers or sisters have had breast cancer. Between 5 and 10 percent of prostate cancer cases are believed to be due primarily to high-risk inherited genetic factors or prostate cancer susceptibility genes, according to the NCI.

Obesity and Weight Gain: A study by the NCI titled "Prospective Study of Adiposity and Weight Change in Relation to Prostate Cancer Incidence and Mortality" shows clearly that obese men are more likely to develop prostate cancer. This large study of 287,000 men is the first to show that weight gain after age eighteen also increases the risk of dying from prostate cancer. During the first six years of the enrollment into the study, 9,986 men developed prostate cancer and 173 died of the disease, according to another NCI study titled "Obesity and Weight Gain Linked to Prostate Cancer Mortality."

BMI category	Percent increased risk of death compared to a person with BMI < 25
Overweight (BMI 25–29.9)	25 percent increased risk of death
Mildly obese men (BMI 30–34.9)	46 percent increased risk of death
Severely obese men (BMI 35)	100 percent increased risk of death

Agricultural pesticide: A long-term study by the National Institutes of Health, National Cancer Institute, National Institute of Environmental Health Sciences, and the Environmental Protection Agency titled "Agricultural Health Study (AHS)" evaluated the role of forty-five pesticides and their possible association with increased prostate cancer risk among pesticide applicators. Methyl bromide was linked to the risk of prostate cancer. Six other pesticides, more often than not found in household products—chlorpyrifos, coumaphos, fonofos, phorate, permethrin, and butylate—were found to increase the risk of prostate cancer among men with family history of the disease.

Screening Procedures

Major medical associations and societies have issued conflicting recommendations regarding screening, making it difficult for an individual to decide if screening is right. The American Cancer Society, American Urological Association, and American College of Physicians recommend that men do the following:

- Consider individual prostate cancer risk factors.
- Know the potential benefits and harms of screening, diagnosis, and treatment.
- Talk to a clinician about concerns or questions.

Several groups recommend men have annual prostate examinations, which should include both a prostate-specific antigen (PSA) blood test and a digital rectal examination (DRE) starting at the following ages:

- by age forty if you are an African-American man or have a family history of prostate cancer or breast cancer
- no later than age forty-five for all other men

Moreover, you should consider the following:

- *Know your PSA.* Keep a record of the exact numbers, not just that it is "in the normal range." Your first PSA blood test typically establishes your baseline PSA score.

- *Track your PSA from year to year.* A rise in PSA levels of 0.75 ng/ml or more within one year may require further investigation by your doctor. The rate of change in your PSA level can be a more significant sign of disease than the actual PSA level.

In addition, the Prostate Cancer Research Institute and several other research centers and prostate cancer specialists recommend a PSA of 2.0 and over at any age should be investigated to rule out prostate cancer.

Screening Tests

Blood Test for Prostate-Specific Antigen (PSA)

PSA is a protein secreted by the epithelial cells of the prostate gland, including cancer cells. An elevated level in the blood indicates an abnormal condition of the prostate gland, either benign or malignant. It is used to detect potential problems in the prostate gland and to follow the progress of prostate cancer therapy.

Free PSA

Free PSA are PSA molecules in the bloodstream that are not bound to other proteins. A free PSA percentage test reports the percentage of free PSA, which is expressed based on free PSA divided by total PSA times 100. One study showed that men with free PSA percentage of greater than 25 percent had low risk, while those with less than 10 percent free PSA were more likely to have prostate cancer.

Digital Rectal Exam (DRE)

A digital rectal exam is a procedure in which the doctor inserts a lubricated, gloved finger into the rectum and feels the prostate through the rectal wall. The prostate is checked for size, hard or lumpy areas, and any pain caused by touching or pressing the prostate. The DRE allows the doctor to feel only one side of the prostate. The test lasts about ten to fifteen seconds.

Transrectal Ultrasound

Transrectal ultrasound can be done in an office, and no sedation or anesthesia is needed. A small probe about the size of a finger is inserted into the rectum and uses sound waves that bounce off the prostate to create an echo. A computer translates these echoes into an image of the prostate. About 80 percent of cancers have an abnormal ultrasound image. Transrectal ultrasound can also help to guide a surgeon to biopsy any area that appears abnormal.

Color Doppler

Doppler imaging helps physicians determine the presence and exact location of a mass within the prostate. Doppler imaging can sense differences in velocity (i.e., blood flow versus solid tissue) and transmit these differences through different color pixels to create a picture on a screen.

PCA3

Recently an additional new screening tool has become available. Bostwick Laboratories now offers the uPM3 test, the first urine-based genetic test for prostate cancer. uPM3 is based on PCA3, a specific gene that is profusely expressed in prostate cancer tissue. On average, the amount of PCA3 is thirty-four times greater in malignant prostate tissue than it is in benign prostate tissue. No other human tissues have ever been shown to produce PCA3. The uPM3 test predicts cancer as confirmed by prostate biopsy with 81 percent accuracy, compared to 47 percent accuracy for PSA. Systematic biopsy of the prostate under ultrasound guidance, however, remains the definitive diagnostic procedure when clinical or laboratory findings indicate the possibility of prostate cancer.

Prostate Biopsy

Prostate biopsies involve excising cores of tissue from the prostate through the rectum. They should not be performed unless there is a persuasive indication that cancer might be present.

The biopsy is usually performed in a physician's office. The patient is positioned in the fetal position, lying on the side with the knees held against the chest. A urologist (a doctor who specializes in treatment of urinary, bladder, and prostate issues) performs the procedure.

Before the biopsy the physician injects the patient with a local anesthetic to numb the skin where the biopsies will be taken (either inside the rectum or at the perineum, the area between the testicles and anus). An ultrasound probe (a thin wand) is inserted into the rectum to locate the prostate and guide the biopsies. A spring-loaded device is used to remove rapidly a one–sixteenth-inch (2.5 mm) by half-inch (20 mm) long cylinder of tissue from the prostate. This is usually repeated twelve times to ensure that tissues from the entire prostate are sampled. The entire procedure usually takes about fifteen minutes. The biopsy samples are then examined with a microscope by a pathologist. The results are usually available within one week.

I underwent a biopsy on my prostate. It was not the first time, but hopefully it will be the last, as I am now considered an ongoing survivor of prostate cancer.

Questions Regarding Prostate Cancer

The time just after I was diagnosed with prostate cancer was a time of conflicting emotions and difficulty in sorting through all the action required and discussions needed with family. When I first started to explore treatment options as well as the experiences of men who had undergone various treatments, I had many questions for my urologist, Dr. Gene Naftulin. I also had questions for the men I interviewed before I made a decision regarding treatment option. My final decision was to be made after a final consultation with my wife and then with Dr. Naftulin, whom I trusted implicitly.

Many men rush into a decision about treatment without first exploring their options and asking the right questions. A few days of hard thinking and soul-searching now may save many problems in the future.

So what were the five most important questions that I chose to ask before I choose a treatment option?

Please note that it is my opinion that at a minimum these questions should be asked of each physician you see. This means you should present questions not only to your urologist and surgeon but also to your radiation oncologist, medical oncologist, and general physician as well.

1. Which treatment option do you recommend, keeping in mind my age, overall health, and stage of cancer?
2. For each treatment option, what are the benefits, costs, and possible side effects I need to be aware of when I am making my decision?

3. What is the likelihood that my cancer will be controlled or cured with each treatment option? What is the likelihood that my cancer will continue to spread with each treatment option?
4. What *side effects or complications* should I expect from each treatment option, and what will these prevent me from doing? Working? Exercising? Enjoying hobbies?
5. If I choose one of these treatment options and it fails to control my cancer, what options would I then have for further treatment?

For me, it was crucial to take the time to ask these five questions as well as several others that my family and I felt were important. In addition, I questioned forty men who had prostate cancer and who had received treatment or watchful waiting in the previous five years. There were different questions I asked of each of them, not the least of which was this: "Given your experience with the treatment that you had and knowing what you know now, would you have the same treatment, or would you opt for a different treatment intervention?"

Side Effects of Prostate Cancer Treatments

Although prostate cancer treatments attempt to destroy only cancer cells, they may also damage healthy cells and tissues. A side effect is an undesirable action or effect of a treatment or drug. The seriousness and duration of side effects vary from patient to patient and depend on the type and extent of treatment.

The treatments for localized prostate cancer—prostatectomy, brachytherapy, and external radiation—have varied side-effect profiles. These should be taken into consideration in the selection of a treatment per a study published online June 9, 2009, in the

Journal of the National Cancer Institute. The treatments for prostate cancer have varying degrees of side effects. The patient should evaluate treatments to decide which one(s) may be most effective and also most suitable for individual preferences and lifestyle.

Many men understand that when prostate cancer is caught early, it can be treated effectively, and the primary treatment options for localized disease are all excellent choices. However, many men also have significant concerns about the side effects of these treatments. The concerns are justified, but there are many misunderstandings about how often side effects occur, how severe they really are, and what can be done to manage them and counteract their occurrence. Many of the side effects men fear most following local treatment are often less frequent and severe than they might think, thanks to technical advances in both surgery and radiation therapy, researchers persistently seeking new ways to help overcome side effects, and improvements in treatment delivery.

It's still important to understand how and why these effects occur and to learn how you can minimize their impact on your daily life. Although doctors plan very carefully for prostate cancer treatment, it is hard to limit the side effects of prostate cancer treatment so that only cancer cells are removed or destroyed. Because treatment also damages healthy cells and tissues, it often causes unwanted and sometimes serious side effects.

There are six broad categories of side effects typically associated with prostate cancer treatments:

- urinary dysfunction
- bowel dysfunction
- erectile dysfunction
- loss of fertility
- side effects of hormone therapy
- side effects of chemotherapy and radiation

There are also a couple of side effects that most men are not informed about before they undergo prostate cancer treatments. These are provided simply to inform you so you can possibly talk about such side effects with your medical specialists.

- *Gynecomastia* (sometimes misspelled as *gynocomastia* or *gynomastia*) is a medical term that means *an abnormal enlargement of the male breast.* It is not unusual for there to be tenderness of the breasts of varying intensity, whether swelling occurs or not. With men undergoing treatment for prostate cancer, it is a *possible* side effect when the amount of testosterone drops through surgery or hormone treatment. It does not occur in all men, and when it does, severity varies widely.
- *Rectal bleeding* is a known complication of one common treatment for prostate cancer, namely external beam radiation. Rectal bleeding can be minimized by use of three-dimensional conformal radiation and by intensity-modulated radiation. If it occurs, remedies are applied to treat it. Because the rectum is close to the prostate, radiation therapy for prostate cancer can injure the rectum's lining. One result may be the abnormal growth of tiny blood vessels near the surface that bleed easily. Studies have shown that between 2 and 20 percent of men who undergo radiation therapy for prostate cancer will develop this condition. Sometimes the bleeding can occur for years following treatment.

Depending on the treatment strategy used, some or all of these side effects might be present. It's also important to realize that not all symptoms are normal and that some require immediate care. Each patient reacts differently. Doctors and nurses can explain the possible side effects of prostate cancer treatment, and they can often suggest ways to help relieve symptoms that might occur during and after treatment. It is important to let the doctor know immediately if any side effects occur.

Late Effects

Late effects of therapy involve unrecognized toxicities that occur many years after therapy.

Knowledge of the possible latent side effects of not only prostate cancer treatments but also other types of cancer therapy can arm survivors with confidence and a plan. By obtaining and incorporating lifestyle interventions, it is possible to reduce the rate of current and late *comorbidities* and adverse therapy-related toxic side effects. Comorbidity is a disease or condition that coexists with a primary disease but also stands on its own as a specific disease.

With the current five-year survival rate at more than 64 percent, the majority of cancer patients will live years and decades longer. Nevertheless, they face various challenges following potential curative or remission therapy, which affect personality, emotions, and social relations. There are also possible physical changes and limitations because of surgery, radiation therapy, chemotherapy, and immunotherapy. Sometimes there may be changes five or ten years after treatment from delayed side effects, such as heart problems following certain therapy. Research is ongoing to evaluate better and safer treatments and also ways of coping and reducing these side effects. In addition, lifestyle changes for improved health are recommended, as most cancer patients die of comorbidities usually related to age, such as complications involving heart, lung, kidney, gastrointestinal, or liver problems.

Those who have had amputations, disfiguring surgery, or colostomies, for example, have effects on daily living activities, self-esteem, and coping. Depression may occur. Often long-term complications from the toxic side effects of therapy not only bring fears and physical problems but also may require specialized treatments and care.

For example, new research shows that patients who receive not only brain radiation therapy but also chemotherapy may have both short-term and long-term memory problems, often referred to as "chemo brain." (The foggy thinking and forgetfulness that cancer patients often complain about after treatment may last for five years or more for a sizable percentage of patients.) The findings, which are based on a study of ninety-two cancer patients at Fred Hutchinson Cancer Research Center in Seattle, suggest that the cognitive losses that seem to follow many cancer treatments are far more pronounced and longer-lasting than commonly believed.

Knowing in advance that this could happen can help reduce anxiety. After appropriate evaluation the patient should be made aware that this is not a recurrence of the cancer but a delayed side effect. Another example of a possible side effect is thyroid failure (hypothyroidism) following neck radiation, which involved the thyroid gland.

Long-Term Effects

Long-term effects are side effects or complications of therapy that persist when therapy is completed, requiring patients to develop compensatory treatment programs to relieve or control these side effects. This is in contrast to late effects, which occur months or years after treatment.

Surgery, radiation, or chemotherapy can cause damage to vital organs, such as the heart, lungs, kidneys, and the gastrointestinal tract. Persons older than sixty-five or seventy may have preexisting heart, lung, kidney, gastrointestinal, or liver problems, which can be accentuated with anticancer therapy, as these organs may be more susceptible to side effects from treatment.

From my own experience with chemotherapy, I have continued to experience *peripheral neuropathy*. Pain, numbness, tingling, or loss of sensation or heat/cold sensitivity in extremities or other areas of the body are often side effects for patients receiving Taxol, Taxotere, platinum, vincristine, Velban, Navelbine, and oxaliplatin drugs.

Cardiac dysfunction problems can occur early or late with treatment of anthracycline drugs, such as doxorubicin (Adriamycin), daunomycin, epirubicin, and mitoxantrone. Long-term follow-up is recommended for possible congestive heart failure up to twenty years and more after treatment. For those who already have cardiac problems, radiation to the heart and treatment with these drugs can also cause progressive cardiac problems. Protective drugs are being developed to delay or prevent damage. In addition, lifestyle changes regarding diet and exercise are important for promoting better health and disease prevention.

Platinum compounds can cause a decrease in kidney function, and this can also be accentuated when there is abdominal radiation involving the kidneys. Platinum compounds can also cause high-frequency hearing loss. For those receiving head radiation therapy, cataracts, dry eyes, and dry mouth are common problems. Abdominal radiation can cause chronic diarrhea, malabsorption, lactose intolerance, bowel dysfunction, and weight loss.

Diagnosis

Granted, prostate exams aren't the most enjoyable things in the
world, but they only last about 10 seconds. It's well worth it.
Just think of the possible consequences if you don't get it done.

—Len Dawson
professional athlete

Being adopted with no biological parent history, I had no
known family history of *prostate cancer*. I was very active and had
no symptoms. My battle with prostate cancer began shortly after I
had surgeries for metastatic melanoma on the top of my head and
in my lymph system in my right neck region. I had come through
those surgeries well and was simply being monitored.

I had a routine physical with my family physician, who
detected some abnormalities in my urine sample. He sent me to
my urologist, Dr. Gene Naftulin. After a thorough examination
in which both a PSA blood test and a DRE were done, the results
indicated an enlarged prostate gland and a significant increase in
my PSA level. In fact, my PSA normal level or baseline was at a
2.7 level and had gradually increased to a 5.0 level when I'd had
my annual physical with my urologist. Now it had doubled less
than a year later. In light of the substantial increase in the PSA
level, my urologist performed a biopsy.

I believe strongly that it is necessary to have one's wife or
significant other as part of the decision-making team with regard
to treatment since the side effects affect both the patient and
spouse. Marty joined me for the consultation with Dr. Naftulin.
He was solemn when he told me, "You have prostate cancer."

We had a thorough consultation with Dr. Naftulin, which
included a frank discussion of the available options, treatment
interventions, and side effects of each. He suggested that I do

some of my own investigation and then discuss the approach I wanted to take. He would not, at that point, suggest one treatment option over another. He wanted me to learn more about the options and consider my choices.

Marty and I left Dr. Naftulin's office without a word spoken between us. We went outside, got into the car, started it, and began driving out of the parking lot. I pulled over, stopped the car, and said, "Oh crap," waited fifteen seconds, and then said, "Okay, now that I am done with self-pity, we will find out all that we can and move forward. This is not going to beat us."

A diagnosis of cancer often causes panic primarily because of a lack of knowledge and fear of the unknown. A patient has options, and members of the prostate cancer community who have "been there, done that" will universally recommend the patient move beyond the panic stage and start to gather knowledge. As I mentioned with regard to my melanoma, knowledge is power. Take your time, do research, and arrive at the best treatment decision for you and your family based on your total health situation.

Medical specialists may steer you in the direction of their specialty and often will understate the risk involved with their treatment of their choice. Urologists tend to favor a surgical option. Surgeons typically favor prostatectomy. Radiation therapists favor radiation, and medical oncologists may focus on androgen deprivation therapy (ADT) and/or chemotherapy. The best choices are made when you have educated yourself with all of the information available.

It must be remembered that any cancer diagnosis and intervention affects others, in particular significant others who are in the patient's circle of close friends and loved ones. A diagnosis of prostate cancer affects a spouse or loved one the most. More often than not, when couples are considering the alternative treatments for prostate cancer, many women say, "I don't care if we cannot have sex again. If it will save his life, I want him to have it (prostate) out!"

As a point of information, if surgery is the chosen approach, there are three ways to remove the prostate. One is the traditional operation through an open incision. The others involve a laparoscope or robot.

Traditional or open surgery for prostate cancer involves the removal of the prostate gland, seminal vesicles, and surrounding pelvic lymph nodes via an incision made between the patient's navel and pubic bone. This highly effective procedure, often called a radical retropubic prostatectomy or simply a prostatectomy, is used to remove prostate cancer completely while preserving the surrounding, unaffected tissue. Physicians commonly perform this procedure with a great amount of focus on the preservation of the nerves and blood vessels that control urination and sexual function. Open radical prostatectomy is a proven method for eradicating prostate cancer.

The word *laparoscopy* means to look inside the abdomen with a special camera or scope. Surgery performed with the aid of these cameras is known as keyhole, porthole, or minimally invasive surgery.

Traditional surgery requires a long incision down the center of the abdomen and a lengthy recovery period. Laparoscopic surgery eliminates the need for this large incision and shortens recovery time.

Other experienced specialists, such as those at Sloan-Kettering Cancer Center and the Sidney Kimmel Comprehensive Cancer Center at Johns Hopkins, have looked at all of the critical variables regarding the different surgical approaches, including blood loss, need for transfusion, pain, erectile dysfunction (ED), cancer cure, side effects related to the surgery, and return to work, and they've found no differences between open surgery or with minimally invasive procedures.

Remember, you are not just choosing a treatment method. You are choosing a doctor. The assets count!

Active treatment usually begins a few weeks to months after diagnosis. A man should meet with doctors, identify the stage and extent of the cancer, discuss treatment possibilities, and find out what survivors in the prostate cancer community have to say about their experiences.

In my case, I interviewed approximately forty men, all of whom had undergone some form of prostate cancer treatment in the past five years, to learn as much as I could about their treatments, the side effects, and implications for quality of life. I asked if, given their overall experience, they would undergo the same treatment. Interestingly for younger men—in their forties and fifties—few would opt again for surgical removal of their prostate, citing a variety of individual reasons. Most expressed disappointment in their sex lives and resultant issues of intimacy. Most indicated that they would have done more research and probably would have chosen another option.

I had several second opinions with various specialists. I met with five different specialists for opinions. One well-known surgeon offered us a "cut-rate" deal, a 20 to 25 percent discount if I paid cash. He could get me in to have my prostate removed within a week. "By the way," he said, "your cancer is a lot worse than what you have been told, so you really need to have this surgery." He had not seen any of the results of the prostate biopsy or other facts in the matter. My wife and I could not get out of there fast enough.

After a consultation with Dr. Daniel Hovenstine, radiation oncologist at Torrance Memorial Medical Center, we made our decision, and then my wife and I met with Dr. Naftulin, who concurred with our choice of treatment.

With prostate cancer, as with other forms of cancer, life is put on hold. This was the case for me, especially since I had been dealing with recent surgeries and related treatments for advanced melanoma. Questions constantly filled my mind. Were the very different cancers related? Had the melanoma cancer cells migrated to my prostate? I wanted to know! Now! My oncologists and specialists calmed my anxiety. No, the melanoma cancer cells had not spread to my prostate. It was pure and simple prostate cancer.

Decision Making

Dr. Hovenstine was patient and thorough. Marty and I had decided on the insertion of radioactive seeds, a form of radiation therapy. (*Brachytherapy* and internal radiation therapy are also terms used to describe this procedure.) However, Dr. Hovenstine explained that though other doctors would probably do such an intervention, he and his colleagues would not. My prostate was too large, and research data had shown that the seeding process would be inadequate to deal with the cancer effectively. There was *no doubt* in my mind that I was in the care of professionals who were competent and caring. Not only did they possess considerable expertise but also displayed considerable concern regarding my safety and health. I was treated like an individual, not a number.

My Treatment

Subsequently we decided to do the intensity-modulated radiation treatment (IMRT). This therapy can be the only treatment given, or it might be prescribed along with surgery and/or chemotherapy. IMRT is an advanced treatment method that allows physicians to target the cancer so effectively that healthy tissue receives little to no radiation, even when the tumor is wrapped around a vital organ.

Once I committed to IMRT and began a treatment schedule, at least once a week I took the staff a box of bagels or other treat. I felt it important to thank them for what they were doing for me, for their caring and giving attitude. It was my way of expressing my gratitude. In addition, typically on Mondays, I would stick my head into the office of the physicist who had the responsibility of making certain that the alignment of the IMRT equipment with my prostate was accurate. I would ask him how his weekend was, if he'd had a good night's sleep, etc. I was acknowledging him as an individual. At one point he told me that no patient had ever looked in on him, joked with him, or brought in any treats. I mention all of this because it was genuine on my part, but it also was intended to help the exceptionally skilled people treat me, to set a gold standard of how I wanted to be treated. I tried to create a personal situation while acknowledging the good work of the staff.

I underwent forty-seven straight days of radiation, with weekends and holidays off for good behavior! The cancer had not spread beyond the prostate. I initially was monitored—checked— at least once every two months and then every three months. Currently it is a semiannual affair.

After my radiation treatments my PSA fluctuated. Though Dr. Hovenstine, my radiation oncologist, indicated that there would be different readings each time my PSA was checked, I had decided that my *score* would be a big fat zero. What a surprise! The first time that my PSA was taken after my radiation treatments, the PSA was a little more than 5.0. I was crestfallen. Dr. Hovenstine was ecstatic. We discussed the findings, and I listened carefully to his explanation about the time frame within which he expected my PSA to move up and down. It was twelve months at a minimum.

The next time he took my PSA it was in the low 3.0 range. More than three years later my PSA was 0.73. My next PSA and consultation will occur in a few months as part of my now semiannual follow-up. As this is written, my PSA has been 0.60 or below.

The most *effective methods* for surviving prostate disease are early screening, knowledge, detection, treatment, and long-term therapy. The biggest piece of advice I can give men is to *become a well-informed prostate cancer patients.*

You can take action to reduce your risk of developing prostate cancer:

- Eat foods conducive to good health in reasonable proportions.
- Follow recommended screening guidelines.
- Exercise regularly.
- Maintain your ideal weight.

Discuss *your* risks with your health-care provider with regard to screening exams, risk-reduction strategies, and the desirable frequency of these testing procedures.

> Once you choose hope, anything's possible.
> —Christopher Reeve
> Actor

> Therefore, choose life!
> —Deuteronomy 30:19

Bibliography

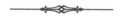

Aggarwal, Bharat B. (corresponding author). "Cancer is a Preventable Disease that Requires Major Lifestyle Changes" in Pharmaceutical Research. September 2008.

American Cancer Society. <http://www.cancer.org/cancer/index>

American College of Sports Medicine. <http://www.acsm.org/>

American Psychological Association. <http://www.apa.org/>

American Society of Clinical Oncology. < http://www.asco.org/>

Association for Applied and Therapeutic Humor. <http://www.aath.org/>

Behar, Diane. "One Patient's Way of Coping, in Cancer Supportive Care Programs." <http://www.cancersupportivecare.com/cope.html>

Benjamin, Harold. The Wellness Community Guide to Fighting for Recovery From Cancer. Putnam Press, 1994.

Bennett, Mary Payne and Lengacher, Cecile. "Humor and Laughter May Influence Health: II. Complementary Therapies and Humor in a Clinical Population." Oxford University Press, 2006.

Cancer Support Community. <http://www.cancersupportcommunitybenjamincenter.org/>

Cancer Support Community, Redondo Beach. <http://www.cancersupportredondobeach.org/>

Caring.com. <http://www.caring.com/>

Carson, Clayborne and Holloran, Peter (editors). A Knock At Midnight: Inspiration from the Great Sermons of Reverend Martin Luther King, Jr. New York: IPM in Association with Warner Books, 1998.

Carson, Clayborne and Holloran, Peter (editors). The Words of Martin Luther King, Jr. New York: Newmarket Press, 1983.

Centers for Disease Control and Prevention. <http://www.cdc.gov/>

Chu-Hui-Lin Chi, Grace, "The Role of Hope in Patients With Cancer," Oncology Nursing Forum, March 2007.

City of Hope Comprehensive Cancer Center. <http://www.cityofhope.org/>

Cleveland Clinic. <http://my.clevelandclinic.org/default.aspx>

Coombs, Arthur Wright (author). Perceiving, Behaving, Becoming: A New Focus for Education. Association for Supervision and Curriculum Development, University of Michigan, 1962.

Cousins, Norman. The Celebration of Life. Bantam Books, 1974.

Cousins, Norman. Anatomy of an Illness. W.W. Norton & Company, 1979.

Cousins, Norman. Head First: The Biology of Hope and the Healing Power of the Human Spirit. Penguin Books, December 1990.

Dana-Farber/Harvard Cancer Center. <http://www.dana-farber.org/>

Dobson, Roger. "How the Power of Touch Reduces Pain and Even Fights Disease." The Independent, Tuesday, 10 October 2006.

Duke University Medical Center. <http://www.dukehealth.org/>

Edman, V. Raymond. Not Somehow, But Triumphantly!, Zondervan Publishing House, 1965.

Emerson, Ralph Waldo. "Nature." The Oxford Companion to American Literature. Ed. James D. Hart. Rev. Philip W. Leininger. Oxford University Press, 1995.

Emerson, Ralph Waldo. "Self-Reliance." <http://www.rwe.org/complete-works/ii---essays-i/ii-self-reliance, Accessed 13 November 2009>

Groopman, Jerome. The Anatomy of Hope. Random House Publishing Group, 2005.

Family Caregiver Alliance. <http://www.caregiver.org/caregiver/jsp/home.jsp>

Fred Hutchinson/University of Washington Cancer Consortium. <http://www.fhcrc.org/en.html, http://www.cancerconsortium.org/en.html>

Habecker, Eugene B. Rediscovering the Soul of Leadership. Taylor University Press, 1996.

Harder, Arlene, "The Nature and Complexity of Hope," http://www.learningplaceonline.com/illness/hope/nature.htm (permission granted by the author, Arlene F. Harder 9/11/2013).

Helldorfer, Martin C. and Moss, Terri. Healing with Heart: Inspirations for Health Care Professionals. Moss Communications, 2007.

Hoffman, Jan. "Doctors' Delicate Balance in Keeping Hope Alive." The New York Times, December 24, 2005.

Journal of Autism and Developmental Disorders <http://www.springer.com/psychology/child+%26+school+psychology/journal/10803>

Journal of Family Nursing. <http://jfn.sagepub.com/>

Kaiser Family Foundation. <http://www.kff.org/>

Kalidasa. Look To This Day (Sanskrit poem). 5th Century AD (because of age of poem, considered as public domain and therefore does not require copyright permission).

Karlin-Neumann, Rabbi Patricia. "Please! Heal! Please! Stanford University Memorial Church, University Public Worship sermon notes, March 18, 2007. <http://www.learningace.com/doc/635128/a68515de2cfc3168d3afab780a19cc65/sermon_03-18-2007_karlin-neumann>

Keltner, Dacher, University of California, Berkeley. Department of Psychology. <http://psychology.berkeley.edu/people/dacher-keltner>

King, Jr., Martin Luther. A Testament of Hope. San Francisco: Harper & Row Publishers, 1986.

Loma Linda University Medical Center. <http://lomalindahealth.org/medical-center/index.page>

Malik, Gretchen. "The Healing Power of Touch." 28 Oct. 2001. 24 Feb. 2009. <http://www.suite101.com/article/cfm/women>

Mayo Clinic Cancer Center. <http://www.mayoclinic.org/departments-centers/mayo-clinic-cancer-center>

McKinney, Kevin. "God's Love can give strength to face our trials." Appears in the Evansville [Indiana] Courier & Press, January 16, 2010 (used by permission of Tim Ethridge, editor, Evansville Courier & Press, 9/9/2013).

Memorial Sloan-Kettering Cancer Center. <https://library.mskcc.org/>

Mandela, Nelson. Long Walk to Freedom: The Autobiography of Nelson Mandela. Little Brown & Co., ISBN 0-316-54818-9 1995.

Moffitt Cancer Center. <http://www.moffitt.org/>

National Cancer Alliance. <http://www.cancersociety.com/>

National Cancer Institute. <http://www.cancer.gov/>

National Cancer Institute's Cancer Information service. <www.cis.nci.nih.gov>

National Institute of Health. <www.cancer.gov>

National Library of Medicine. <http://www.nlm.nih.gov/medlineplus>

Oakwood Cancer Care Center. <http://www.oakwood.org/cancer-care>

Oncology Nursing News. <http://www.onclive.com/>

Parachin, Victor M., in **American Fitness**, "The Healing Power of Touch: The Simple Act of Touching Frequently

Reduces Everyday Anxiety and Tension," November-December 1991. (Used by permission of Tom Ivicevic, publisher, American Fitness magazine, 9/22/2013.)

Poon, Leonard W. and others. "Understanding Centenarians' Psychosocial Dynamics and Their Contributions to Health and Quality of Life." Current Gerontology and Geriatrics Research, Volume 2010 (2010).

Psychology Today. <http://www.psychologytoday.com/>

Rayel, Michael G., First Aid to Mental Illness: A Practical Guide for Patients and Caregivers, Soar Dime, 2002, 2008.

Rustøen, Tone, (and team). "The importance of hope as a mediator of psychological distress and life satisfaction in a community sample of cancer patients." Centre for Shared Decision Making and Nursing Research, Oslo University Hospital, Rikshospitalet, Norway. Cancer Nursing July-August, 2010.

Saint John's Health Center
<http://www.newstjohns.org/home.aspx>

Sasson, Remez. Visualize and Achieve. Remez Sasson, 2004.

Siegel, Bernie. Love, Medicine & Miracles. HarperCollins Publishers 1986. ISBN 0-06-091406-8, ISBN 978-0-06-091406-6

Smedes, Lewis, Standing on the Promises. Thomas Nelson Inc. 1998.

Spiro, Howard and Yale University Program for Humanities in Medicine. The Power of Hope: A Doctor's Perspective. New Haven [Conn.]: Yale University Press, 1998.

Stanford Cancer Institute. < http://cancer.stanford.edu/>

Taylor University. <http://www.taylor.edu/>

The Angeles Clinic and Research Institute.
<http://www.theangelesclinic.org/>

The Holy Bible. The University Press, Cambridge, King James
Version (KJV), 1949, (also Revised Standard Version (RSV),
New International Version (NIV), New Revised Standard
Version (NSRV).

The National Cancer Institute Cancer Information service.
<www.cis.nci.nih.gov>

The National Coalition for Cancer Survivorships.
<http://www.canceradvocacy.org/>

The National Library of Medicine – Medline.
< http://www.nlm.nih.gov/medlineplus/>

The Sidney Kimmel Comprehensive Cancer Center,
Johns Hopkins.
http://www.hopkinsmedicine.org/kimmel_cancer_center/

The Ohio State University Wexner Medical Center.
<http://medicalcenter.osu.edu/Pages/index.aspx>

Thiboldeaux, Kim and Golant, Mitch. The Total Cancer
Wellness Guide. BenBella Books, Inc., 2007.

Torrance Memorial Medical Center.
<http://www.torrancememorial.org/>

Touch Research Institute.
<http://www6.miami.edu/touch-research/>

University of California Los Angeles Jonsson Comprehensive
Cancer Center. <http://www.cancer.ucla.edu/>

University of Pennsylvania Cancer Center.
<http://www.penncancer.org/> and
<http://www.oncolink.org/index.cfm>

University of Southern California Norris Comprehensive
Cancer Center. <http://ccnt.hsc.usc.edu/>

University of Texas MD Anderson Cancer Center.
<http://www.mdanderson.org/>

Wellstar Health System.
<http://www.wellstar.org/pages/default.aspx>

World Cancer Research Fund.
<http://www.wcrf.org/index.php>

World Health Organization. <http://www.who.int/en/>

Yale University School of Medicine.
<http://medicine.yale.edu/index.aspx>